State of the World's Vaccines and Immunization

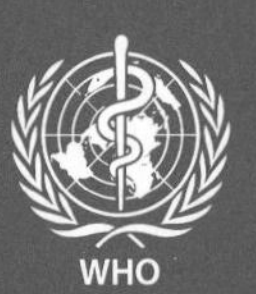

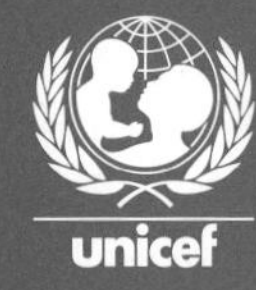

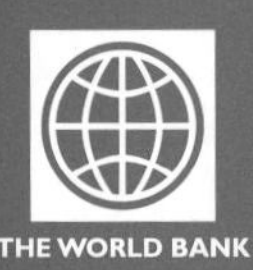

Acknowledgements

State of the World's Vaccines and Immunization

We wish to dedicate this book to the many health workers, scientists, volunteers, and civil servants whose lives have been dedicated to vaccine development and immunization, some of whom have lost their lives in the accomplishment of their work.

Acknowledgements and contributions

Writer: Sheila Davey

Editor: Mick Geyer

Initial research: Becky Owens

Editorial Board: Mahenau Agha, Yagob Almazrou, Amie Batson, James Cheyne, Peter Folb, Heidi Larson, Jean Marie Okwo Bele, Daniel Tarantola, Michel Zaffran

Special thanks for their critical help to: Diana Chang Blanc, Ulli Fruth

Administrative Assistance: Pankaj Bhayana, Silvia Kirori, Kreena Govender

Contributors and reviewers: Teresa Aguado, Isao Arita, Ray Arthur, Bruce Aylward, Louise Baker, Norman Baylor, Julian Bilous, Lahouari Belgharbi, Yves Bergevin, Maureen Birmingham, Claire Broome, Steve Brooke, Michael Brennan, Brent Burkholder, Tony Burton, Center for Biologics, Evaluation and Research at the US Food and Drug Administration, Claire-Lise Chaignat, Karen Chaitkin, Thomas Cherian, Children's Vaccine Programme at the Programme for Appropriate Technologies in Health, Gaël Claquin, John Clements, Mario Conde, Laura Cooley, Alya Dabbagh, Robert Davis, Claudia Drake, Philippe Duclos, Nedret Emiroglu, Howard Engers, Sarah England, Jose Esparza, Evidence and Information for Policy Cluster of WHO, Carl Frasch, Jackie Fournier-Caruana, Marta Gacic-Dobo, Taky Gafaar, François Gasse, Shawn Gilchrist, Roger Glass, Hana Golding, Tracey Goodman, Marion Gruber, David Gwatkin, Anamaria Henao-Restrepo, Carol Hooks, Annemarie Hou, International Federation of Pharmaceutical Manufacturers Associations, Bernard Ivanoff, Héctor Izurieta, Pal Jareg, Luis Jodar, Gareth Jones, Mark Kane, Umit Kartoglu, Marie-Paule Kieny, Dennis Kopecko, Ulla Kou, Steve Landry, Gordon Larsen, Barbara Lautenbach, Rune Lea, Pat Leidl, Mike Levine, Ruth Levine, Jon Liden, Andrei Lobanov, Patrick Lydon, Marty Makinen, Lewis Markoff, Jacques-François Martin, Marcelle-Diane Matsika-Claquin, Raymond Mbouzeko, Susan McKinney, Christine McNab, Bjørn Melgaard, François Meslin, Roeland Monasch, Karen Midthun, Julie Milstien, Violaine Mitchell, Germano Mwabu, Carib Nelson, Chris Nelson, Gus Nossal, Jean Marc Olivé, Sonia Pagliusi, Gordon Perkin, Judy Ranns, Alison Rowe, Bryn Sakagawa, Suomi Sakai, Claudia Stein, Hiro Suzuki, Ingvar Theo Olsen, Michel Thuriaux, Jos Vandelaer, Jay Wenger, Jerry Weir, Roy Widdus, Scott Wittett, Lara Wolfson, Kathy Zoon.

Contents

Acronyms

AAVP	African AIDS Vaccine Programme
AD	Autodisable syringes
ADIP	Accelerated development and introduction plan
AIDS	Acquired immunodeficiency syndrome
BASICS	Basic Support for Institutionalizing Child Survival
BCG	Bacille Calmette-Guerin (existing TB vaccine)
CDC	Centers for Disease Control and Prevention
CRS	Congenital rubella syndrome
DNA	Deoxyribonucleic acid
DOTS	Directly Observed Treatment Short Course
DR Congo	Democratic Republic of Congo
DT	Diphtheria-tetanus vaccine
DTP	Dipththeria-tetanus-pertussis vaccine
DTwP	Diptheria-tetanus-(whole cell) pertussis vaccine
EPI	Expanded Programme on Immunization
ETEC	*Enterotoxigenic Escherichia coli*
FIOCRUZ	Oswaldo Cruz Foundation (Brazil)
GMP	Good Manufacturing Practices
GAVI	Global Alliance for Vaccines and Immunization
GNP	Gross National Product
Hib	*Haemophilus influenzae* type b
HIPC	Heavily Indebted Poor Countries
HIV	Human immunodeficiency virus
HIV/AIDS	Human immunodeficiency virus/ Acquired immunodeficiency syndrome
HPV	Human papillomavirus
HSV-1	Herpes simplex virus type 1
HSV-2	Herpes simplex virus type 2
IAVI	International AIDS Vaccine Initiative
ICC	Interagency Coordinating Committee
ICG	International Coordinating Group
ICGEB	International Centre for Genetic Engineering and Biotechnology
IFRC	International Federation of Red Cross and Red Crescent Societies
IDA	International Development Association
IDRI	Infectious Disease Research Institute
IPV	Inactivated polio vaccine
MMR	Measles-mumps-rubella combination vaccine
MR	Measles-rubella combination vaccine
MVI	Malaria Vaccine Initiative
NCI	U.S. National Cancer Institute
NGOs	Nongovernmental organizations

NIDs	National Immunization Days
NIH	National Institutes of Health
NIAID	National Institute of Allergy and Infectious Diseases
NRA	National Regulatory Authority
OPV	Oral polio vaccine
PAHO	Pan American Health Organization
PATH	Program for Appropriate Technology for Health
PFP	Purified F protein
R&D	Research and development
RBM	Roll Back Malaria
RRV-TV	Rhesus rotavirus vaccine-tetravalent
RSV	Respiratory syncytial virus
SIGN	Safe Injection Global Network
SIV	Simian immunodeficiency virus
SHIV	Chimeric SIV/HIV
SOS	Sustainable Outreach Services
SVDP	Schistosomiasis Vaccine Development Project
SWAP	Sector Wide Approach
TB	Tuberculosis
TDR	UNDP/World Bank/WHO Special Programme for Research and Training in Tropical Diseases
TT	Tetanus toxoid
UNAIDS	Joint United Nations Programme on HIV/AIDS
UNDP	United Nations Development Programme
UNFPA	United Nations Fund for Population Activities
UNICEF	United Nations Children's Fund
USAID	U.S. Agency for International Development
VVM	Vaccine vial monitor
WHO	World Health Organization

Foreword

Imagine a world without vaccines. Life-threatening diseases would present a daily risk. We would live in fear of deadly strains of diphtheria, tetanus and measles; polio would be a constant danger and in a matter of hours could paralyze a child, and smallpox would continue to scar and kill. All these diseases would claim the lives of our children in vast numbers, families watching helplessly. Lives would be cut short and people's movement severely restricted. Cities would be places to flee at the first rumour of infection rather than magnets for culture, commerce and learning. It is hard to imagine the loss in lives, creativity, productivity, potential and well-being.

This is not an imaginary place or a description of the past. For many people in our world – most of them poor – this is still the reality. Immunization, as powerful and successful as it is, has yet to reach its enormous potential. One-quarter of the world's children still have no protection from common preventable diseases. Nearly 3 million people (2 million of them children) die every year from those same killers. Children in developing countries are dying from other diseases, such as meningitis and pneumonia, while vaccines for these are widely used in the industrialized world.

The world needs to address gaps in immunization services in both rich and poor countries. The right to protection from preventable diseases is the right of every child and it is well within our collective capacity to realize that right. We must ensure that every child benefits from one of the most cost-effective health interventions available, and that all children are vaccinated safely, effectively and equitably.

In public health terms we are compelled to act. Infectious diseases such as HIV/AIDS and tuberculosis are threatening our economic and social stability. Epidemics spread faster and further than ever before. Our health interdependence has deepened. Immunization in one country is the key to reduction of disease in others. We all have a role to play as guardians of health: as leaders in countries, agencies and corporations, responsible for furthering political, economic, social and research agendas; as parents once children ourselves.

Together we can find new vaccines to stop the worst killer diseases, and ensure that existing vaccines are taken out of the laboratory and put into the field – to reach every child. Together we truly can deliver a 'global public good', a benefit for all, regardless of national borders, by making a concerted effort to use the tools that medically promise so much. Immunization remains one of the best investments in health that is within our grasp. We have a responsibility that we cannot ignore.

Gro Harlem Brundtland
Director General, WHO

Carol Bellamy
Executive Director, UNICEF

James Wolfensohn
President, World Bank Group

Call to action

Immunization has been a great public health success story. The lives of millions of children have been saved, millions have the chance of a longer healthier life, a greater chance to learn, to play, to read and write, to move around freely without suffering. Smallpox has been eradicated, other diseases are better controlled, children's rights have been acknowledged and laws to protect them enacted and enforced. Soon we will make history again. Polio, once a global epidemic, will be eradicated; a further reminder of what immunization can do. It is the most powerful of all preventive health measures for children and it is central to human rights and poverty alleviation. It is the right of every child to be given this kind of protection.

But as this report tells us, these advances have not come fairly to all children in all places. More and more children are being systematically excluded depending on where in the world they live.

Children are our future, they are our best hope, their suffering our worst fear. Parents the world over will lie awake at night with fears and dreams in equal measure for what lies ahead for them. Our actions can help or hinder their development. With the resources that the world has at hand, it is possible to break the cycles of poverty and disease. Starting with immunization, we can reduce the inequities of our world and tackle today's major epidemics, like HIV/AIDS, so that the next generation has an equal chance of life and health.

Guardians of health, we urge you to take up this challenge: we call on governments and civil groups, organizations of the United Nations system and nongovernmental organizations, philanthropists and responsible corporate citizens, to recognize immunization as a global public good. Meet your moral and financial commitments to the world's children and make a greater investment in immunization. You are already forming new alliances, already taking great strides, already making bold changes. We urge you, who hold the key to a healthy future, to work together each day to fulfil your duty – and there can be none more important – to protect the health and welfare of all children and uphold the rights of those who trust us and depend on us to show them the way.

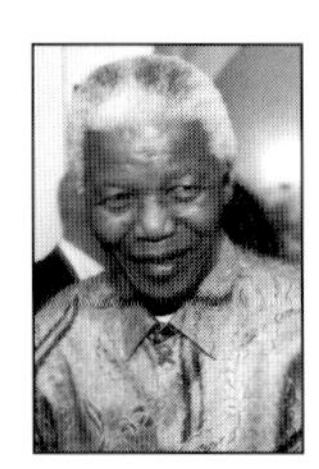

Nelson Mandela
Chair – Vaccine Fund Board

Executive summary

Overview

This latest edition of *State of the World's Vaccines and Immunization* highlights the immense strides made in global immunization since the mid-1990s. These include the near-eradication of polio worldwide as well as dramatic reductions in the incidence of measles and maternal and neonatal tetanus in some of the lowest-income countries. This report also charts progress in the development and introduction of new life-saving vaccines that have the potential to save millions of lives every year.

However, the report also points out that many children have yet to benefit from these achievements. While some low-income countries have made substantial progress in increasing immunization coverage, coverage in others is at its lowest for over a decade. In sub-Saharan Africa, for example, only about 50% of children are immunized during their first year of life. By contrast, the wealthier developed countries have not only far higher immunization rates but children also have access to a wider range of vaccines.

Part 1 of this report charts the growing divide in access to vaccines and immunization and warns of the global consequences of failure to sustain investments in immunization in developing countries. These include the re-emergence of diseases that were once under control, the spread of diseases to countries and continents where they had been eliminated, and the immense social costs of disease in the countries worst affected.

Part 2 outlines new initiatives launched in response to mounting international concern at low immunization coverage, the growing inequalities in immunization and the unacceptable toll of infectious diseases in developing countries. The aim of these initiatives is to improve access to underused vaccines, accelerate the discovery and introduction of priority new vaccines, catalyze new sustainable financing and raise both political commitment and public demand for immunization.

Part 3 looks at the impact of some vaccines already in use today and reviews progress in the research and development (R&D) of priority new vaccines for developing countries.

Part 4 outlines some of the reasons why the world community should invest in immunization and looks at the promising future for vaccines and immunization.

Immunization challenges

Immunization, together with improvements in hygiene and sanitation, has revolutionized child health in countries throughout the world, preventing millions of deaths every year in addition to reducing the risk of disability caused by infectious diseases.

Through national immunization programmes around the world, millions of deaths have been prevented every year since the launch of the Expanded Programme on Immunization (EPI) in 1974. Smallpox was eradicated in 1979, a massive human endeavour, and today polio is set to become another scourge of the past.

However, the wider benefits of immunization are not reaching all children. In some of the least-developed countries, children have less access to immunization services than those in wealthier countries. In some cases, children lose out because immunization services suffer from low political commitment and under-investment. The poorest children typically have access to a smaller range of vaccines and are at greater risk from the hazards of unsafe immunization practices. These problems are compounded by low levels of investment in the research and development of new vaccines urgently needed in developing countries.

While global **immunization coverage** of over 70% was sustained throughout the 1990s, this achievement masked wide variations both between and within countries. In some developing countries, immunization rates increased substantially. But elsewhere, especially in sub-Saharan Africa, immunization rates plummeted, leaving millions of children vulnerable to life-threatening childhood diseases. Meanwhile, in Europe, the political, economic and social changes that followed the demise of the former Soviet Union, triggered a dramatic decline in immunization rates in many countries in East and Central Europe and the newly independent states. By 2000, approximately 37 million children worldwide did not receive routine immunization during their first year of life (see Fig.1, p. xv).

Inequalities also exist between the poorest and wealthiest populations within countries, with the highest inequalities in countries that are both poor and have low overall rates of immunization coverage. Not surprisingly, the poorest 20% of the world's population suffer significantly greater proportions of infectious diseases and other conditions. Their children account for over half of all childhood deaths from pertussis, polio, diphtheria, measles and tetanus, and for 45% of all deaths from perinatal conditions.

In some developing countries, efforts to meet immunization targets are hampered by poorly functioning **health service delivery systems**. In countries where health services barely exist outside urban areas governments are often unable to meet the basic health needs of the population. Elsewhere, buildings, vehicles and vital cold chain equipment may be poorly maintained or in disrepair, and the ability to deliver health services, including immunization, may be compromised by weak managerial skills, poor motivation of staff, and a failure to plan and budget effectively. In addition, the lack of effective disease surveillance and reporting systems in some developing countries undermines the effectiveness of immunization and disease control programmes and makes it difficult to target health services to those in greatest need.

Meanwhile, **inequity in access to new vaccines** has increased over the past two decades as new life-saving vaccines have become available at prices that most low-income countries have been unable to afford. However, lack of funds has not been the only barrier. Until recently, many of the poorest countries lacked the capacity to deliver existing vaccines, let alone add newer, more expensive ones such as the hepatitis B and *Haemophilus influenzae* type b (Hib) vaccines. Furthermore, the inadequacy of disease surveillance and reporting systems in some countries has made it difficult to establish both the burden of disease and the potential cost-effectiveness of any of the new vaccines.

However, low or uncertain demand for a new vaccine at the outset can have a long-term impact on both the supply and price. Faced with low and/or uncertain demand in developing countries, manufacturers will limit the scale of production accordingly. And once manufacturing plant size has been established, it is very expensive to scale up production at a later stage. Therefore, the low volume of production further ensures that prices are likely to remain relatively high.

Gaps also exist in the **R&D** of new vaccines. Despite major breakthroughs in the development of new vaccines over the past twenty years, the needs of children in developing countries are not being addressed by vaccine R&D agendas tailored to the needs of children in wealthier countries.

The low uptake of new vaccines in developing countries has also been a major disincentive for manufacturers to invest in new vaccine R&D. In addition, the low prices negotiated over the years for traditional vaccines such as diphtheria-tetanus-pertussis (DTP), polio, measles and tuberculosis (BCG), for use in developing countries have deterred vaccine manufacturers from developing vaccines for particular use in what are perceived to be "low profit" countries. Vaccine manufacturers therefore, have little commercial incentive to develop vaccines against diseases such as HIV/AIDS, TB and malaria, which kill millions of people in developing countries but relatively few in the developed world.

An additional constraint is that new vaccines against diseases that occur in developed countries are often not suitable for use in developing countries. The same disease may be caused by a different type of organism in developing countries and may take a completely different, often more dangerous form, especially among children also suffering from malnutrition.

The report also draws attention to the failure of some developing countries to pay sufficient attention to **immunization safety**. Until recently, some countries were unable to guarantee the quality and safety of the vaccines used in their immunization programmes. Elsewhere, children's lives have been needlessly put at risk by unsafe injection practices.

All vaccines that are prequalified by WHO for supply through UNICEF and other UN agencies conform to WHO regulatory standards, including those for good manufacturing practices (GMP). However, not all countries have a fully functioning and effective national regulatory authority with the capacity to guarantee the **quality and safety of vaccines**. This applies to both those that are produced domestically as well as those that are imported. Vaccines that have not been manufactured and tested to appropriate standards can do harm. Furthermore, those that do not meet potency standards may fail to protect children against the targeted diseases.

In addition, the potency and safety of vaccines is sometimes compromised by programme errors. The training and supervision of product handling, transportation, storage and safe administration are necessary in order to ensure safe and effective vaccines.

Lives may also be put at risk by failure to ensure **injection safety**. While in the developed countries problems are largely restricted to injecting drug use and occasional needle-stick injuries among health workers, in the less-developed countries unsafe injection practices are rife and account for an estimated US$ 535 million in health care costs and 1.3 million deaths a year.

However, injections for immunization account for less than 10% of all injections for medical purposes and are generally considered to be safer than curative injections, which include many unnecessary and unsafe injections. Other issues of importance to injection safety include the sterilization of equipment, waste disposal and training, each of which are discussed later in this report.

Meanwhile, **immunization funding** has failed to keep up with population growth and the higher cost of delivering services. In some cases, absolute funding levels have fallen dramatically over the past decade due to withdrawal of donor support and greater pressure on public spending. Consequently, routine immunization programmes have been neglected in some developing countries.

Although immunization is one of the State's core public health responsibilities, many governments in low-income countries are not able to allocate adequate and reliable financial resources to immunization. The least-developed countries, which, even after donor support, spend on average only US$ 6 per capita a year on all health services, including immunization, are unable to mobilize the resources needed to expand coverage. Even in developing countries with a relatively higher national income, immunization programmes suffer from funding uncertainties, competition from both within and outside the health sector, and increases in funding requirements as coverage expands and new vaccines become available. Overall, developing countries are achieving significantly less of the benefits of immunization. The rich-poor immunization gap will continue to grow, if left to domestic government resources alone.

Charting a way forward

In response to mounting international concern at low immunization coverage, the growing inequalities in immunization, and the unacceptable toll of infectious diseases in developing countries, new global partnerships have been forged to break the cycle of neglect. Foremost among these is the Global Alliance for Vaccines and Immunization (GAVI, also known as The Alliance), which brings together major stakeholders in immunization from both the public and private sector: WHO, UNICEF, the World Bank Group, national governments, international development banks, bilateral agencies, nongovernmental organizations (NGOs), the Bill & Melinda Gates Foundation, the Children's Vaccine Program at the Program for Appropriate Technology for Health (PATH), foundations, public health programmes, and representatives of the vaccine industry from both developing and developed countries. Together these partners offer a broad range of skills including vaccine research, production, supply, immunization programme delivery, international financing mechanisms, advocacy and communications.

Launched in early 2000, the Alliance aims to increase coverage with new and existing vaccines and accelerate the R&D of priority vaccines for use mainly in developing countries.

The Alliance operates through a new financing mechanism, the Vaccine Fund, established with an initial grant of US$ 750 million over five years from the Bill & Melinda Gates Foundation, and boosted to US$ 1 billion by contributions from the governments of Canada, Denmark, the Netherlands, Norway, Sweden, the United Kingdom, the United States and private contributors. The goal of the Alliance is to raise US$ 2 billion over five years.

Progress so far has been dramatic. Within two years, 90% of the low-income countries eligible for support had applied for assistance through the Vaccine Fund. Five-year grants totalling over US$ 800 million have been awarded to 54 countries, including war-torn countries such as Afghanistan, Liberia and Sierra Leone, in addition to three populous countries: China, India and Indonesia. The GAVI partners estimate this investment will help increase basic immunization rates in funded countries by 17% and boost coverage with hepatitis B vaccine from 18% to 65% by 2007 – potentially preventing over 2 million deaths.

New initiatives have also been launched to ensure the **R&D** of priority vaccines for developing countries. The public sector needs to do far more to estimate the burden of disease, forecast demand and guarantee a market for new vaccines at affordable prices in developing countries. A firm commitment upfront to purchase safe and effective vaccines will reduce the risk for vaccine manufacturers of uncertain demand and help re-direct global research towards the vaccines that are a priority for developing countries. In addition, predictable market conditions can help secure the availability and affordability of new vaccines through credible demand forecasts, bulk purchasing schemes and futures agreements.

Efforts are also under way to strengthen the capacity of developing countries to carry out **clinical trials** of priority vaccines. Only a limited number of research centres exist with the capacity and experience needed to conduct large-scale clinical trials of new vaccines, which can involve tens of thousands of people over several years. As a result, progress is stalled on some of the vaccines already in the pipeline and urgently needed in developing countries. In order to ensure progress on this issue, the public sector needs to work in partnership with vaccine manufacturers to build the capacity needed in developing countries for applied vaccine research, clinical evaluation and early introduction of priority new vaccines.

Meanwhile, **recent trends in the vaccine market** are likely to have an impact on both the supply and price of vaccines for use in developing countries. Over the past decade, a series of mergers between some of the major pharmaceutical companies, coupled with the shrinking manufacturing base for low-profit traditional vaccines, has resulted in a global shortage of some vaccines. The reduction in the number of suppliers to the global market has made vaccine supply increasingly vulnerable to lot failures, further contributing to recent vaccine shortages.

While new vaccine development is today carried out mainly by large multinational manufacturers based in developed countries, developing country manufacturers are already playing a major role in manufacturing and are expected to play an increasing role in product development in the future. By 2000, 50% of UNICEF's vaccine procurement, even without taking polio vaccine into account, was purchased from these so-called "emerging producers". In addition, several developing country manufacturers have entered into joint agreements with major vaccine manufacturers for the production of some vaccines.

Another recent phenomenon is the increasing divergence between vaccine schedules in high-income and low- and middle-income countries, which could have an impact on both the supply and price of vaccines for use in developing countries. This development involves both the introduction of new vaccines to meet the needs of developed countries (e.g. pneumococcal and meningoccocal conjugate vaccines, based on the forms of the bacteria that circulate in developed countries), and the development of new vaccine substitutions to meet the increased regulatory requirements of the developed countries. Examples of vaccine substitutes include acellular pertussis vaccine to replace the whole cell pertussis component of DTP vaccine and inactivated polio vaccine (IPV) to replace live oral polio vaccine (OPV), while whole cell pertussis vaccine and OPV remain the vaccines of choice in developing countries. Furthermore, the removal of the mercury-based preservative thiomersal from vaccines, in response to recommendations from regulatory bodies in the developed countries, has resulted in a switch to more expensive single-dose vaccine vials for developed country markets which has placed greater demands on manufacturing capacity, thereby increasing the fragility of the vaccine supply chain.

The section on **improving immunization services (Part 2, section 3)** highlights efforts to strengthen immunization services and health service delivery systems in developing countries.

Countries that apply for funding support through GAVI are being offered funding and capacity building support. This support is contingent on countries carrying out an overall assessment of their immunization services, using a set of agreed standards, to identify both their strengths and weaknesses. On the basis of this, countries establish a multi-year plan of action for immunization, in addition to making commitments to meet targets for strengthening any weak links in the system and for raising coverage. Furthermore, national governments and development partners are being urged to ensure that immunization services are central to health sector development plans and that immunization targets are used as key performance indicators for development.

Efforts are also being intensified to reach increasing numbers of children with immunization. To achieve this, countries are being encouraged to introduce district-level monitoring and performance targets. This gives a truer picture of immunization coverage than national averages which can conceal huge disparities between rich and poor, as well as between urban and rural settings.

In countries where there is no recognizable health infrastructure or where health services barely exist outside urban areas, immunization is being used to build a bridge to the poorest children as well as those who are hardest to reach. By putting children on the health planner's map through immunization, the possibility for other contacts, such as micronutrient supplements and routine health checks, can add further benefits to these programmes.

Meanwhile, new global initiatives have been launched to promote and monitor immunization safety standards and support the development of safer vaccine technologies.

In 1999, WHO forged a new global partnership aimed at improving immunization safety worldwide. The Immunization Safety Priority Project brings together national governments, UNICEF, UNAIDS, the World Bank Group, the Children's Vaccine Program, PATH, industry, development agencies and professional organizations. By 2003, it aims to ensure the safety of all immunizations as well as the safe management of waste disposal. The immunization safety priority project also participates in the Safe Injection Global Network (SIGN) alliance, established in 1999 to ensure the safe and appropriate use of all injections worldwide.

Also in 1999, WHO established an independent panel of experts in vaccine safety to advise on all vaccine safety issues. The Global Advisory Committee on Vaccine Safety also assesses the implications of vaccine safety issues for vaccine practices worldwide as well as for WHO policies. To date, the committee has considered more than 20 major safety issues with potential implications for global immunization policy.

WHO has trained key health personnel responsible for national immunization policies and vaccine regulation on issues including vaccine safety, monitoring and dealing with vaccine-related adverse events, and how to deal openly and fully with the media on vaccine safety issues.

Since the mid-1990s, WHO has been involved in efforts to strengthen the capacity of national regulatory authorities (NRAs) to assess the **quality and safety of vaccines** used within a country – whether domestically produced or imported from elsewhere. The aim is to ensure that all countries have access to vaccines of assured quality and that the quality is maintained up to the time the vaccine is administered.

In 1996, a Global Training Network was established to provide training in the regulation of vaccines for staff from NRAs, national immunization programmes and vaccine manufacturers. And since 1997, regular assessments have been carried out by teams of experts to determine whether the NRA is performing a set of essential regulation functions for vaccine. WHO has also developed guidelines and training courses for health workers to ensure that immunization safety procedures are correctly followed and minimize the risk of programme errors.

Efforts to improve **injection safety** have also been stepped up. In 2000, a joint statement was issued by WHO, UNICEF, UNFPA, and the International Federation of Red Cross and Red Crescent Societies (IFRC) urging all donors who finance vaccines to supply all vaccines together with autodisable (AD) syringes (designed to prevent re-use) and puncture-proof safety boxes for safe waste disposal. They also recommended that standard disposable syringes and needles should no longer be used for immunization and that the use of sterilizable syringes should be phased out by 2003. In addition, countries applying for support through GAVI are required to develop an injection safety plan as part of their application to the Vaccine Fund. WHO has also produced guidelines on the management of health care waste, including injection equipment.

The section on **financing vaccines and immunization** (Part 2 section 4) underlines the critical need to increase the financing of immunization in developing countries and looks at a range of potential new financing mechanisms.

National governments in both developing and developed countries have the primary responsibility to assure the sustainable financing of their national immunization programme. However, as routine immunization coverage has fallen in many of the poorest countries and newer vaccines remain out of reach for many of the children who need them most, there is a growing consensus that increased financing of immunization is also a shared global responsibility.

GAVI partners are working with governments to increase the level of funding available, while taking steps to avoid the aid dependency that characterized the 1980s. Governments are being encouraged to take on a coordinating role. They are being urged to assume overall responsibility for securing sustainable funding for their vaccine needs from both domestic and external resources, and for using those resources as efficiently as possible. In return for external support, they are also required to meet standards for quality and safety, to reach increasing numbers of hard-to-reach children, and to take steps to ensure sustainable financing. This new approach depends on strong government commitment to immunization, backed up by good evidence (e.g. estimates of the cost-effectiveness of vaccines compared to other health interventions) in order to argue the case powerfully with decision-makers.

Towards a brighter future

Vaccines hold great promise for the future. New vaccines already exist that have been proven both safe and effective. The problem is that they are often unavailable where they are needed most. But there is now greater understanding within the public sector of the vaccine production cycle and of what is needed to break this deadlock. This includes:

- Efforts to better understand and overcome the constraints experienced by existing manufacturers in making vaccines more affordable
- Defining the most cost-effective options for vaccine manufacture for developing countries, including increased vaccine manufacturing capacity in these countries
- Building capacity in countries to optimize the impact of vaccines and reduce wastage
- Ensuring creative and sustainable financing mechanisms and well-coordinated procurement plans
- Advocating for more equitable access to priority vaccines, both new and old, for children who need them most.

With adequate investment there is renewed hope that the promise of immunization can be realized for children throughout the world. The GAVI partners are today providing the catalyst needed to reverse the decline in immunization, accelerate the introduction of new vaccines in developing countries and anchor immunization at the heart of development efforts. In addition, other organizations and development partners around the world are working to put an end to the unacceptable status quo in immunization in order to establish a new, more equitable system for the world's children.

Figure 1: **Children not immunized (DTP3), 2001 (in millions)**

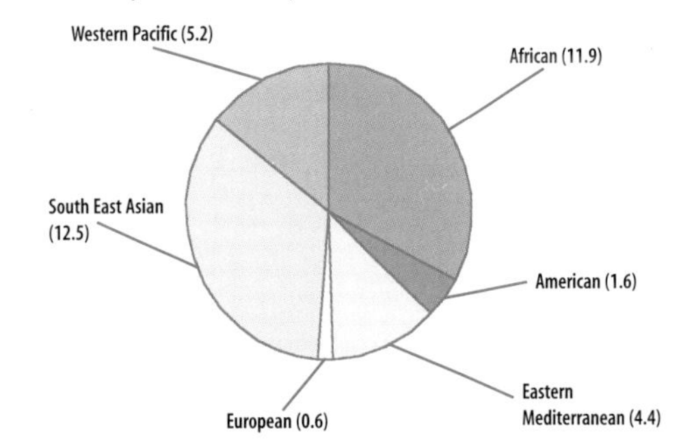

Source: Best Estimates WHO/UNICEF, 2002

Part 1:
Immunization challenges

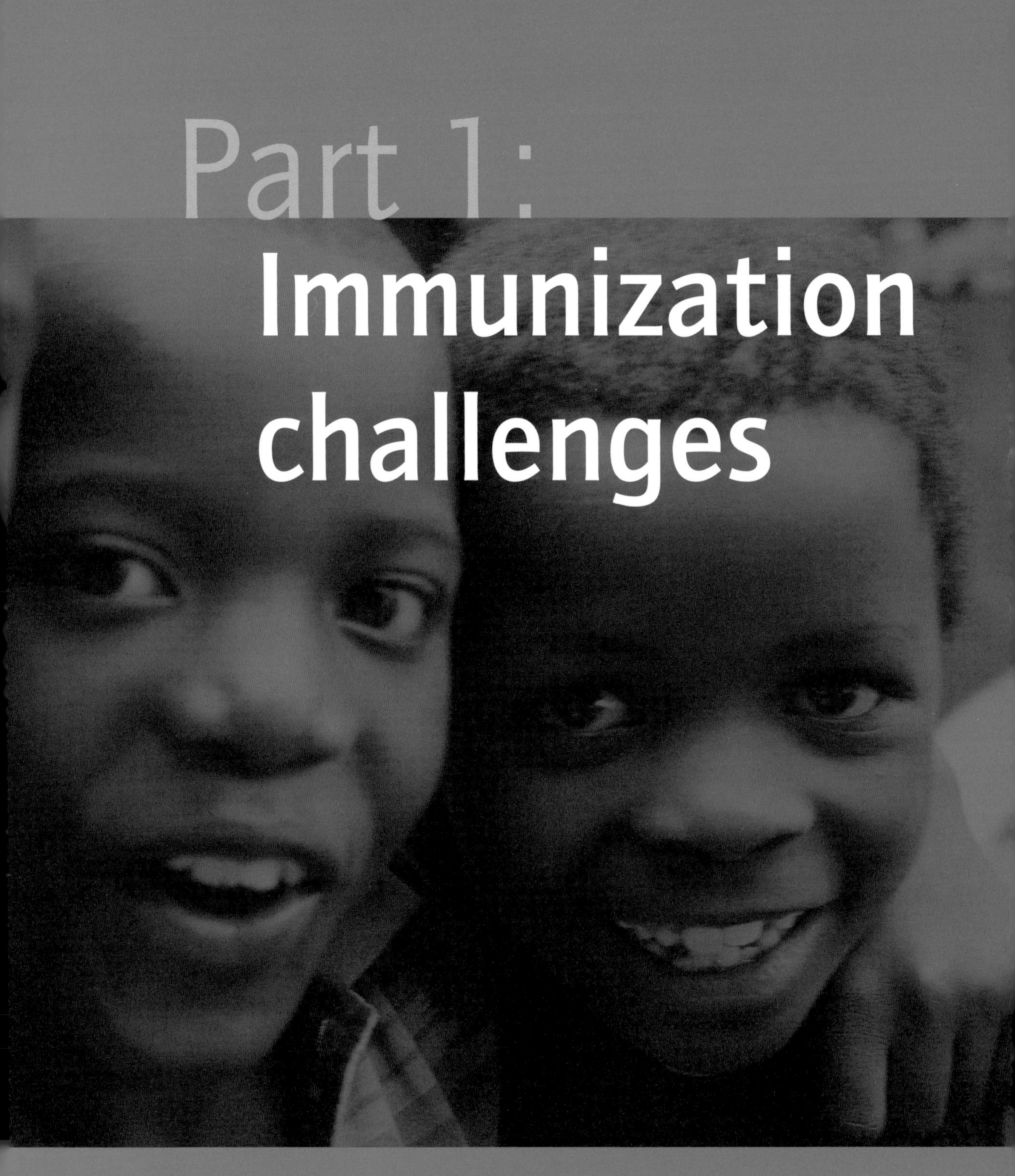

vaccin

Part 1 of this report highlights the gaps that have opened up in access to vaccines and immunization. It focuses on inequity in the following areas:

- immunization coverage
- access to health services (including immunization)
- access to new vaccines
- vaccine research and development
- immunization safety
- the financing of immunization programmes.

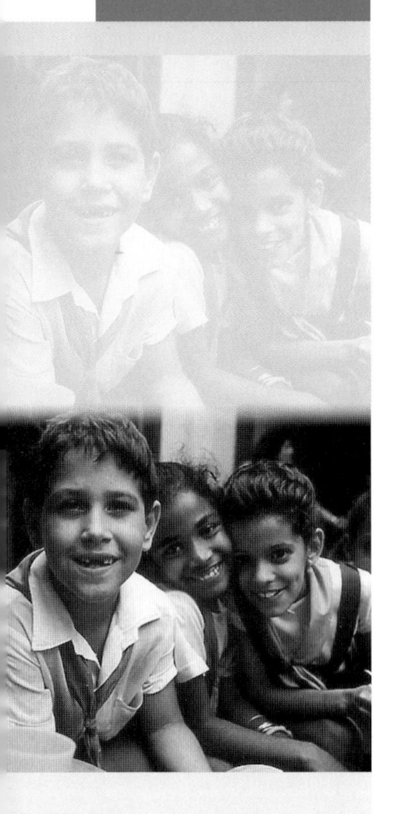

Immunization, together with improvements in hygiene and sanitation, has revolutionized child health in countries throughout the world, preventing millions of deaths every year and reducing the risk of disability caused by infectious diseases. Today, immunization is one of the most cost-effective ways of improving health and of opening up access to other vital health interventions such as nutritional supplements or malaria prevention.

However, the promise of immunization has not been fulfilled for all children. In some of the least-developed countries, children have less access to immunization services than those in wealthier countries. The poorest children typically have access to a smaller range of vaccines and are at greater risk from the hazards of unsafe immunization practices. Immunization services in developing countries may suffer from low political commitment and under-investment, while immunization programmes are hampered by weak health service delivery systems. These problems are further compounded by low levels of investment in the R&D of new vaccines that are urgently needed in developing countries.

1. Coverage gaps

This section looks at the gaps in immunization coverage that have opened up not only between countries and regions but also between the poorest and wealthiest populations within individual countries.

Immunization has prevented millions of deaths every year

Immunization stands out as one of the greatest public health achievements of the twentieth century. Through national immunization programmes around the world, millions of deaths have been prevented since the launch of the Expanded Programme on Immunization (EPI) in 1974. Smallpox was eradicated in 1979, polio is about to be eradicated and about two-thirds of developing countries have succeeded in eliminating neonatal tetanus.

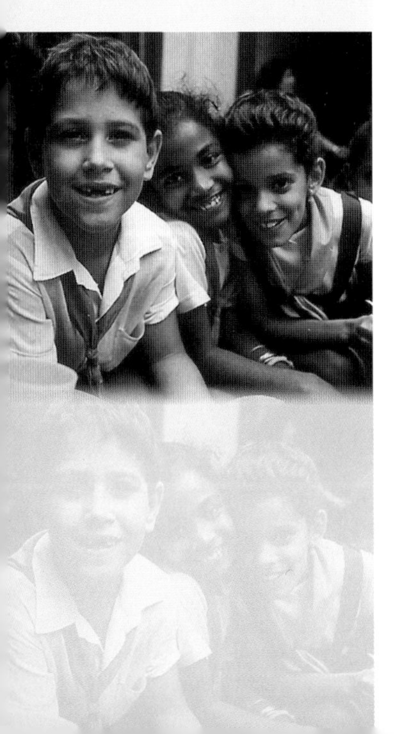

But global commitment to immunization has not been sustained in all developing countries. In some low-income countries, less than one in three children are immunized during their first year of life. By 2000, about 37 million children worldwide missed out on routine immunization during their first year of life. Today, the divide in access to vaccines and immunization continues to undermine the principle of equity on which national immunization programmes should be based.

Despite the overall success of immunization programmes, almost 11 million children under five years of age die each year. Immunization with existing vaccines could prevent many of those childhood deaths as well as reducing the toll of disability, illness and missed schooling among the children who survive.

While global immunization coverage of over 70% was sustained throughout the 1990s, (see Fig 2), this global average masked wide variations both between and within regions. In sub-Saharan Africa, for example, immunization rates peaked at 55% in 1990 and remained at about the same level throughout the 1990s. By 2000, only 53% of children in this region were immunized with DTP, the vaccine that protects against diphtheria, tetanus and pertussis (whooping cough).

Meanwhile, regional averages can also conceal wide variations in immunization coverage in individual countries. In some developing countries – notably Bangladesh and Latin American countries including Bolivia, Brazil, El Salvador and Nicaragua – immunization rates increased substantially. But in other low-income countries, especially in sub-Saharan Africa, childhood immunization rates plummeted, leaving millions of children vulnerable to life-threatening vaccine-preventable childhood diseases.

In Somalia, which has one of the lowest immunization rates in the world, only 18% of children were fully immunized with DTP. In Nigeria, the most populous country in Africa, less than one in four were vaccinated. Yet only a decade earlier, more than twice as many children had been immunized. Similar declines were reported in the Central African Republic (from 82% in 1990 to 29% in 2000) and in Congo, (from 79% to 33% over the same period).

Elsewhere, in Europe, the break-up of the Soviet Union, and the political, economic and social changes that ensued triggered a dramatic decline in immunization rates. In many countries in east and central Europe and the newly independent states, immunization rates plummeted leading to the re-emergence

Figure 2: **Immunization coverage, 1980–2001, 3 doses DTP – global and by region**

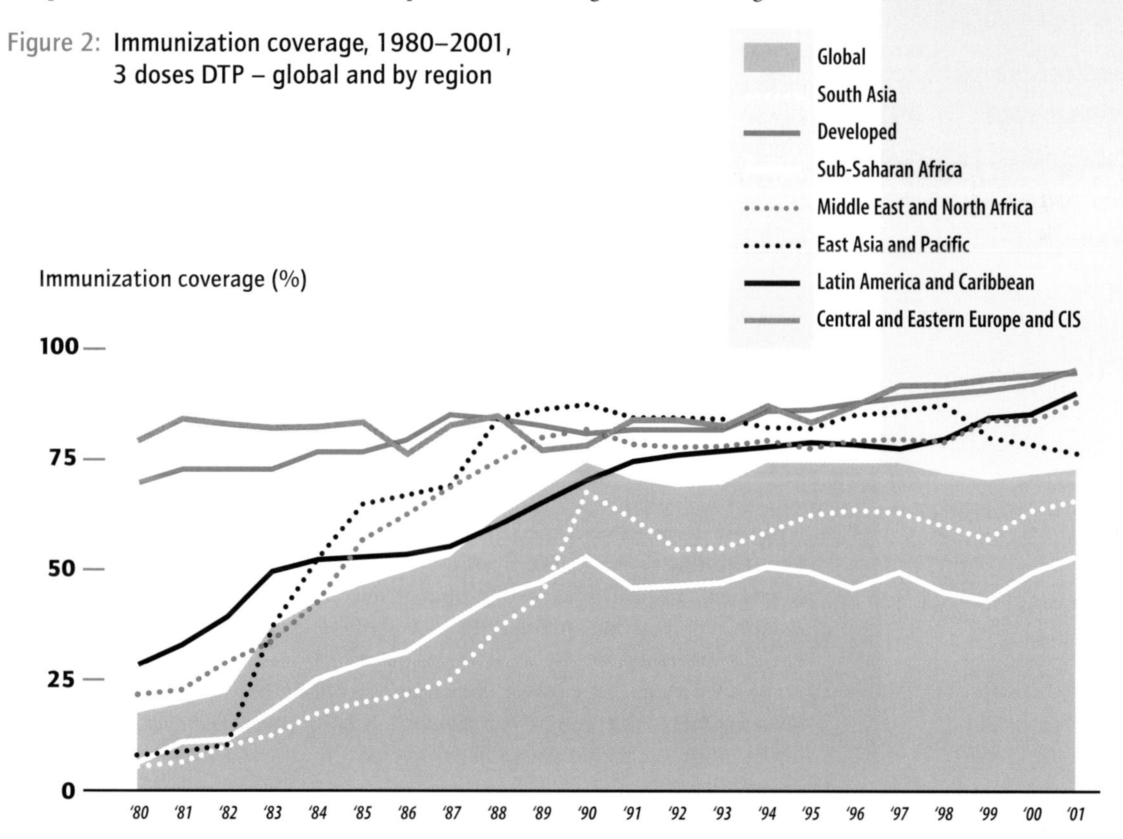

Source: Best Estimates WHO/UNICEF 2002

of diseases such as diphtheria. Many countries were unable to ensure adequate supplies of vaccines and could not afford the cost of establishing safe and efficient vaccine delivery systems. As a result, great disparity exists today between the vaccines available in the high-income countries of Europe and those with economies in transition.

Meanwhile, in developing countries throughout the world, children miss out on immunization because they are trapped inside conflict zones or living in remote areas beyond the reach of any health services. Others are excluded because their parents fail to register their birth or make use of health services even where they exist.

Although the annual number of measles cases declined by almost 40% globally during the 1990s, in many countries measles immunization coverage is dangerously low, particularly in sub-Saharan Africa and South Asia. In 2000, about 770 000 children died from measles worldwide, mainly in developing countries, more than any other vaccine-preventable disease. A highly contagious disease, measles can rapidly spread among children who have not been immunized. In 1998, 1400 children died in a single outbreak of measles in an area along Lake Kivu in the war-torn Democratic Republic of Congo.

Low immunization rates and outbreaks of disease pose a serious threat to non-immune children and adults in all countries worldwide

Maternal and neonatal tetanus are also vaccine-preventable diseases that mainly affect the poor. Although more than 100 developing countries have succeeded in eliminating neonatal tetanus, it remains a public health problem in 57 developing countries. In 2000, 200 000 newborn babies died from neonatal tetanus. These deaths occurred because their mothers were not fully immunized against the disease (and therefore could not pass on their immunity) and due to a lack of hygiene during or after the birth. Mothers who are fully immunized can protect their babies against tetanus during the first two months of life, up to the age when they themselves can be immunized against the disease. About 30 000 women also die every year from tetanus infection after giving birth. In some of the poorest countries, fewer than one in three women of childbearing age have been immunized with tetanus toxoid (TT).

While global immunization coverage rates largely reflect the huge gap in health status between the poorest and wealthiest countries, inequalities also exist between the poorest and wealthiest populations within countries. Recent studies by the World Bank reveal that within many countries immunization rates are consistently higher among the wealthiest groups. And that the highest inequalities are in countries that are both poor and have low overall rates of immunization coverage, mainly in sub-Saharan Africa. In Niger, where the divide is greatest, the wealthiest 20% of children are ten times more likely to be immunized than the poorest 20%. Elsewhere, in Côte d'Ivoire, India and Nigeria, for example, the wealthiest children are four times more likely to be immunized than the poorest. In addition, immunization drop-out rates are highest among the poorest populations, who may fail to complete the full immunization schedule due to limited access to, or irregular provision of health services.

The poorest 20% of the world's population are more susceptible to infectious diseases and other conditions, due to a wide range of reasons, including malnutrition, low provision of health services and the cost of medicines. Their children account for over half of all childhood deaths from pertussis, polio, diphtheria, measles and tetanus, and for 45% of all deaths from perinatal conditions.

At the Millennium Summit held in New York in September 2000, a set of eight Millennium Development Goals (MDGs) were established and agreed by UN member states. The fourth goal, to reduce child mortality, has the specific target of reducing under-five mortality by two-thirds between 1990 and 2015. One of the specific indicators to measure progress towards the goal is the proportion of one-year-old children immunized against measles. In 2001, the United Nations Development Programme (UNDP) estimated that over 60% of the population in developing countries were in states that were "lagging, far behind, or slipping" in meeting the MDGs for reducing child mortality rates. In sub-Saharan Africa, for example, deaths among children under five almost doubled over the past four decades from 2.3–4.5 million a year. In this region, out of every six mothers who give birth today, at least one will lose her child before their fifth birthday, often during the first month of life. Millions more children are growing up with no protection against some of the life-threatening, disabling and vaccine-preventable diseases of childhood.

We the Children
End-decade review of the follow-up to the World Summit for Children

Report of the Secretary General – May 2001

"Immunization continues to be one of the most practical and cost-effective public health interventions. The levelling-off of immunization coverage during the 1990s is due primarily to:

- A failure in some countries to secure domestic and international resources for immunization;
- A lack of protection for financing of immunization services during some health sector reforms, at least temporarily;
- The inability of some public health systems to fully reach very poor families, minorities and those living in remote locations-and the impact of conflicts on others;
- A failure to fully exploit the potential of National Immunization Days (NIDs) as a supplement to immunization programmes.

Immunization systems in many developing countries are still fragile and of uneven quality. There are growing concerns about the safe administration of injectable vaccines. These challenges will need to be addressed if today's opportunities for large-scale introduction of new and improved vaccines are not to be missed."

Meanwhile, low immunization rates and outbreaks of disease pose a serious threat to non-immune children and adults in all countries worldwide. The rapid growth in international travel and mass population movements have increased the potential for diseases to spread, not just across national borders but to other continents as well. As health interdependence has deepened, immunization in one country can affect the prevalence of disease in another. Many of the explosive disease outbreaks of the past decade have occurred far from the original source of infection.

In the early 1990s, an international health emergency was declared in Eastern Europe when low immunization rates and economic crisis triggered a major epidemic of diphtheria in which 30 000 people died. By the time the epidemic had been brought under control, the disease had also spread to Finland, Germany, Norway and Poland. And, in 1996, the importation of an Asian strain of poliovirus (most probably from India or Pakistan) sparked an outbreak of the disease in Albania, which later spread to neighbouring Kosovo and Greece.

2. Health service delivery gaps

This section highlights the difficulty in meeting immunization targets in countries with poorly functioning health service delivery systems where governments are unable to meet the basic health needs of the population.

Failure to ensure routine immunization for children is not only due to a lack of sustained funding for immunization. It is also the result of poorly managed and poorly equipped health service delivery systems, which, in some low-income countries, is the result of decades of under-investment and neglect.

In some countries, health services barely exist outside urban areas, while elsewhere, buildings, vehicles and vital cold chain equipment may be poorly maintained or in disrepair. Vaccine safety may also be compromised by storage in ill-functioning refrigerators and freezers, or when sterilizing equipment breaks down and contaminated syringes and needles are rinsed in tepid water, then re-used.

Meanwhile, the ability to deliver health services, including immunization, may also be compromised by weak managerial skills, poor motivation of staff and a failure to plan and budget effectively. In addition, the lack of effective disease surveillance and reporting systems undermines the effectiveness of immunization and disease control programmes and makes it difficult to target health services to those in greatest need. In some countries, communications and infrastructure are so poorly developed that the majority of the population have no access to health services, let alone immunization.

In some countries, conflict has destroyed infrastructure and fractured health service delivery systems. In 1999, for example, only 18% of children were fully immunized with DTP in Somalia, while in Ethiopia and Chad only 21% were fully immunized. Meanwhile, public health systems in sub-Saharan Africa generally, are overwhelmed by the increasing burden of HIV/AIDS. This problem is further exacerbated by HIV-related illnesses, absenteeism and deaths among health workers. In 2001, UNAIDS reported that some countries were losing one-quarter of their health workers to AIDS. In one hospital in Zambia, deaths among health workers increased thirteen-fold between 1980 and 1990 – largely due to HIV/AIDS.

In 2000, a WHO study on human resources in public health systems, *Human Resources for Health*, highlighted an alarming mismatch in some countries between the health needs of the population and the geographical location of health workers, the size of the workforce and the mix of skills available. Some of the 18 countries involved had an oversupply of graduate doctors and nurses, while others had severe shortages of qualified staff. Countries in Africa reported an overall shortage of health workers - the result of limited training capacity and low pay - while most countries cited a severe shortfall of health personnel in rural areas. In Angola, for example, only 15% of health workers work in rural areas, where an estimated 65% of the population live. However, this problem is not specific to Africa. In Cambodia, for example, 85% of the population live in rural areas but only 13% of health workers are based there.

Meanwhile, health workers complained of low pay and few benefits, a lack of basic amenities such as electricity and clean water, and poor working conditions (e.g. inadequate facilities, shortages of equipment and essential drugs, and having to work in conflict zones). In such circumstances it is not altogether hard to understand why many developing countries may have difficulties in recruiting and retaining health personnel.

3. Gaps in access to new vaccines

This section outlines some of the reasons why, until recently, developing countries have been unable to access new life-saving vaccines. It points out that unless developing countries are able to estimate the impact of disease and the cost-effectiveness of a new vaccine, demand will remain low or at best uncertain – with major implications for both the long-term supply and price of the vaccine.

The divide in access to vaccines between wealthy and poorer countries has widened even further over the past two decades

The divide in access to vaccines between wealthy and poorer countries has widened even further over the past two decades (see Fig. 3), as new life-saving vaccines have become available – at prices that most low-income countries could not afford. However, lack of funds is only part of the problem. In many of the poorest countries, immunization systems lacked the capacity to deliver existing vaccines, let alone add new, more expensive ones. In addition, the inadequacy of disease surveillance and reporting systems in some countries made it difficult to establish the burden of disease and the potential cost-effectiveness of any of the new vaccines. As a result, immunization schedules differ in low-, medium- and high-income countries – with the wealthier countries including a wider range of antigens (see Annex 3).

However, lack of demand for a new vaccine at the outset can have a long-term impact on both the supply and price. Faced with low or uncertain demand in developing countries, manufacturers will limit the scale of production accordingly. And once plant production size has been established, it is very expensive to scale up production at a later stage. In addition, the low volume of production ensures that prices are likely to remain relatively high.

Figure 3: Number of childhood vaccines routinely used in developing and established market countries

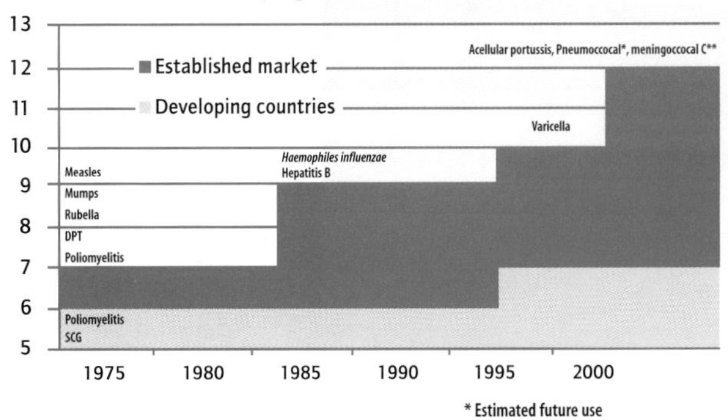

* Estimated future use
** Used in – 50% of global birth cohort
Source: WHO

The following case illustrates this point. In the developed countries the widespread use of Hib vaccines against *Haemophilus influenzae* type b (a strain that causes some forms of pneumonia and meningitis) almost eliminated Hib-related diseases over the past decade. However, during the same period, many developing countries did not have the capacity to establish the burden of Hib disease, in addition to the fact that the vaccine was initially too expensive for most low-income countries to contemplate. As a result, an estimated 4.5 million unvaccinated children died from Hib-related diseases, mainly pneumonia, in developing countries in the same 10-year period.

Hepatitis B vaccine, the first cancer-preventing vaccine, has shared a similar fate since it first came on the market in 1981. Despite a massive reduction in price from US$ 150 at the outset to under US$ 1-1.5 today for a three-dose course, the vaccine still costs almost as much as all six original EPI vaccines combined. Over 520 000 people die from hepatitis B infection every year due to acute hepatitis B infection and chronic infection (leading to cirrhosis and liver cancer). In 1992, WHO recommended that every national immunization programme should introduce the vaccine by 1997, but this target is far from being met. By 2001, 72 countries were still not using the vaccine in their routine immunization programme.

In 2000, a report by the International AIDS Vaccine Initiative (IAVI), declared that the customary long wait for the introduction of new vaccines in developing countries was "a colossal public health failure." The report warned that a delay of even five years in the introduction of a future AIDS vaccine in low-income countries could result in up to 30 million needless HIV infections.

4. R&D gaps

This section highlights under-investment in the research and development of new vaccines urgently needed in developing countries. Low profit margins for traditional children's vaccines and low uptake of new vaccines in developing countries have deterred vaccine manufacturers from investing in new vaccines for mainly low-income countries. The problem is compounded by differences in the prevalence of disease-causing organisms in developing and developed countries.

Despite major breakthroughs in the development of new vaccines over the past two decades, children in developing countries are disadvantaged by vaccine R&D agendas tailored to the needs of children in wealthier countries. The problem is three-fold: first, the low uptake of new vaccines in developing countries; second, the neglect of "low-profit" vaccines for mainly developing country markets; and third, differences in the prevalence of disease-causing organisms in developing and developed countries.

Low or uncertain demand for new vaccines in developing countries, together with the low prices negotiated over the years for the traditional six vaccines (DTP, polio, measles and BCG) for use in developing countries, have deterred vaccine manufacturers from developing vaccines for use almost exclusively in what are perceived to be "low profit" countries.

Vaccine R&D is an increasingly risky, lengthy and costly business, and uncertain demand for a new product is one of the major risk factors for a vaccine manufacturer. Each new vaccine can cost US$ 500 million or more to research and develop, often over a period of 12–15 years. In order to recoup these costs and make a profit, vaccine manufacturers subsequently set a high price for each new vaccine. Exclusive rights to an initial 20-year period following the introduction of the vaccine is protected by patents under the Agreement on Trade Related Aspects of Intellectual Property Rights (also known as the TRIPS agreement).

Patents give the manufacturer exclusive rights to either produce the vaccine themselves or license production to another manufacturer in return for payment of royalties. Once the patents have expired, other vaccine manufacturers are free to produce the vaccine without payment of royalties. Over time, this leads to competition, which in turn may lead to over capacity and a willingness to sell at a low profit margin. In the meantime, millions of children's lives are being lost in developing countries, where governments are unable to afford the new vaccines until the price is reduced, 10–20 years later (see Fig. 4 below).

Today, vaccine manufacturers have little commercial incentive to develop vaccines against diseases such as HIV/AIDS, TB and malaria, which kill millions of people in developing countries but relatively few in the developed world. For example, of the approximately US$600 million a year invested in HIV vaccine

Figure 4: **Average vaccine development costs per product**

	Pre-clinic	Phase 1	Phase 2	Phase 3	Pre-registration	Registration	LAUNCH →
Years	2.4	2.0	1.8	1.4	1.1	1.3	10
Market entrance probabilities %	22	39	54	68		98	YEARS
**Number of candidates in pipeline*	4.6	2.5	1.9	1.5		1***	
***Cost of drug development/candidate US$ m*	8.5	12	33	39			
Cost of vaccine development/candidate US$ m Year 2000	5–7	6–9	37–68	46–48		30–40***	

* n= 591 candidates between 1993 and 1994

** For large pharmaceutical firms $>360 million sales

*** Additional post marketing trials has increased regulatory and licensing costs in line with Phase 3 trials

Source: Struck, M., Vaccine; Vol. 14 pp. 1,301_1,302, 1998

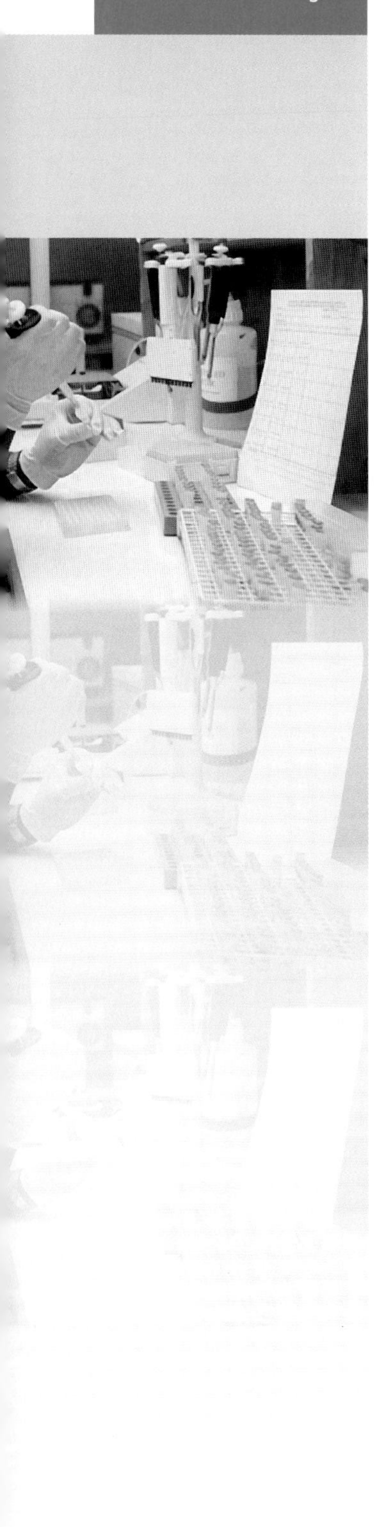

research, the majority comes from the US National Institutes of Health (a public sector institution). To put that amount in perspective, in 1999, research spending on drugs to treat HIV/AIDS was about US$ 3 billion in Europe and the United States alone. Other diseases fare just as badly. In the 1996 report *Investing in Health Research and Development,* WHO highlighted some of the distortions in global health research funding. At the time of the study, acute respiratory infections, diarrhoeal diseases and TB – which together account for almost 8 million deaths a year, mainly among the poor – attracted an estimated US$ 99 million–133 million (0.2% of the total amount spent on health research including vaccine R&D). By contrast, more was spent on research into asthma – an estimated US$ 127 million–158 million – which accounts for 218 000 deaths a year worldwide.

An additional constraint for vaccine R&D is that new vaccines against diseases that occur in developed countries are often not suitable for use in developing countries. The same disease may be caused by a different type of organism in developing countries and may take a completely different and often more dangerous form, especially among children also suffering from malnutrition. In the United States, for example, a new vaccine is now routinely used to protect young children against pneumococcal disease. But the new vaccine is not appropriate for use among children in developing countries – where pneumonia caused by pneumococcus is a major cause of death among children under five – because it offers no protection against two key serotypes of the bacterium that are widespread in developing countries but not found in the United States.

A similar setback for developing countries was the decision by vaccine manufacturers in the late 1990s to halt development of a new conjugate vaccine against serogroups A and C meningococcal meningitis and switch to other potentially more profitable combination vaccines instead. In the developed countries, a new conjugate vaccine is available to protect children against serogroup C meningococcal disease (the most frequent cause of epidemics in these countries). But since the abandonment of the serogroup A/C conjugate vaccine, no conjugate vaccine has been developed to protect children in developing countries against serogroup A meningococcal meningitis – which can occur in explosive epidemics, often with major loss of life. In the United Kingdom, which started using the serogroup C meningococcal vaccine in 1999, there were less than 20 cases of the disease in 2000. In 1996, an epidemic of serogroup A meningococcal disease in the so-called Africa "meningitis belt" (which stretches from Ethiopia in the east to Senegal and the Gambia in the west) involved at least 200 000 cases and claimed about 20 000 lives – the worst meningitis epidemic on record.

Likewise, HIV vaccine research remains heavily skewed towards the development of a vaccine for developed country markets, where infection rates appear to have slowed down. Of the US$ 500 million a year spent on vaccine development, only about US$ 40 million is being used to develop a vaccine to protect people in developing countries – where 95% of infections occur.

5. Immunization safety gaps

This section highlights the failure of some developing countries to pay sufficient attention to immunization safety. It points out that until recently some countries were unable to guarantee the quality and safety of the vaccines used in their immunization programmes. Elsewhere, as a result of unsafe injection practices, children's lives have been needlessly put at risk

Vaccine quality and safety

All vaccines that are prequalified by WHO for supply through UNICEF and other UN agencies (see Annex 1 on prequalified vaccines page 85) conform to WHO regulatory standards, including those for Good Manufacturing Practices (GMP). However, in some developing countries, the quality and safety of the vaccines used cannot be guaranteed. This compromises the effectiveness of immunization programmes and puts children's lives at risk.

Problems can arise at different stages: during the vaccine production process; during the transportation and storage of the product; and, for some vaccines, during the reconstitution process, when it is mixed with a liquid (diluent) before being administered.

Not all countries have a fully functioning and effective national regulatory authority with the capacity to guarantee the quality and safety of either domestically produced or imported vaccines. In 2001, of the 48 countries which were vaccine producers, over 60% met WHO standards for a fully functional national regulatory authority. However, of over 60 countries that imported vaccines (other than vaccine pre-qualified by WHO for supply through UNICEF), only about 16% were able to guarantee the quality and safety of the vaccines used. Vaccines that have not been manufactured and tested to appropriate standards can do harm, while vaccines that do not meet potency standards may fail to protect children against the targeted diseases.

In the late 1990s, for example, evidence emerged of a fake meningitis vaccine that contained no active ingredients, but which was supplied during an outbreak of the disease in Niger. Without an adequate regulatory authority, fake vaccines and inappropriately manufactured vaccines can slip through the net. As a result, both children and adults may die from the very diseases the counterfeit vaccines were supposed to prevent.

In addition, the potency and safety of vaccines may be compromised by programme errors in some developing countries. Inadequate training and supervision of product handling, transportation, storage and safe administration, can lead to the administration of a vaccine that is neither safe nor effective.

In the past, children's lives have been put at risk by programme errors including undetected breaks in the cold chain (the critical cold storage network of refrigerators, freezers and cold boxes) and use of vaccine beyond its expiry date.

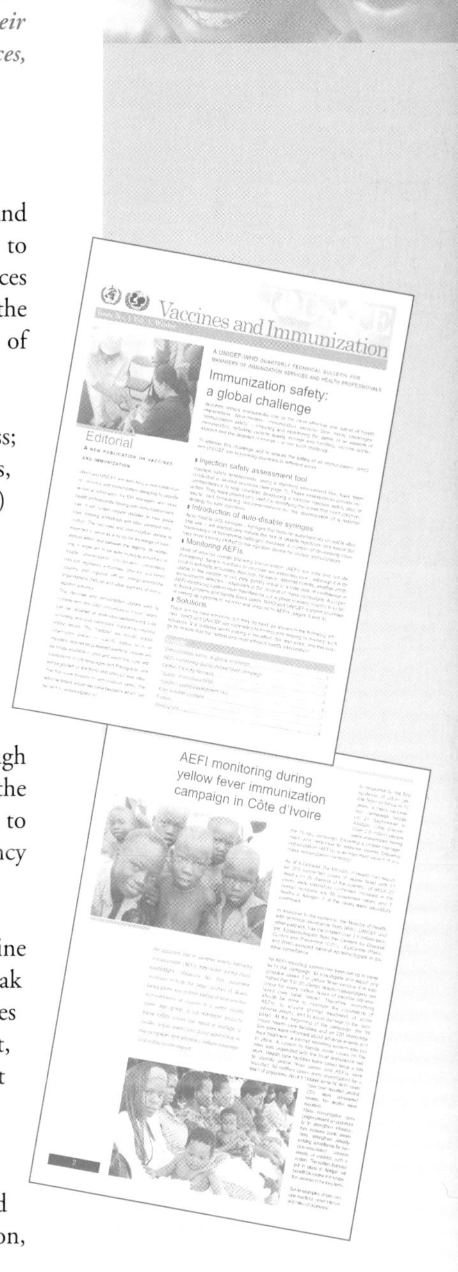
Vaccines and Immunization

Immunization safety: a global challenge

Editorial

Injection safety assessment tool

Introduction of auto-disable syringes

Monitoring AEFIs

Solutions

AEFI monitoring during yellow fever immunization campaign in Côte d'Ivoire

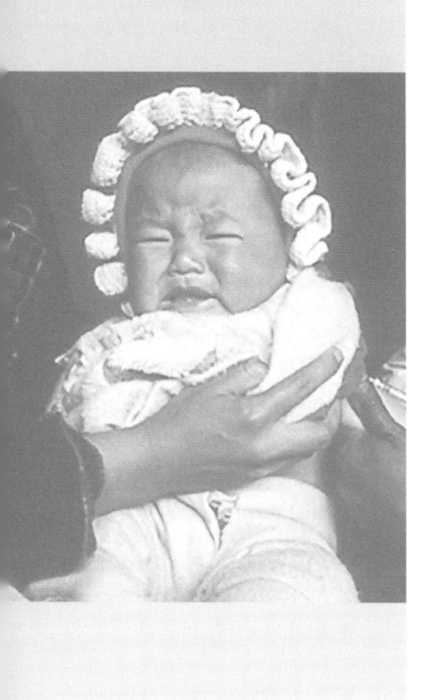

Another potential hazard is the reconstitution of vaccines such as measles which have to be mixed with a diluent before use. In several instances, health workers have inadvertently used a drug instead of a diluent and children have died, or children have been given a vaccine which failed to protect them because too much diluent had been added by mistake. In addition, children's lives have also been put at risk from bacterial infections when reconstituted vaccine that should be thrown away after each immunization session – so as to avoid the risk of contamination – has been stored overnight and re-used.

In developing countries, programme errors, rather than the vaccine itself, are the most common cause of Adverse Events following Immunization (AEFI)*. Without a rapid and effective response to any of these potential problems, public confidence in immunization evaporates overnight, immunization coverage drops and outbreaks of disease occur, often with disastrous consequences. However, not all developing countries have effective surveillance systems in place with the capacity to rapidly detect, investigate and respond to immunization problems as soon as they arise.

By contrast, in the developed countries, the receding threat of infectious diseases has focused attention on the relative risk from the vaccine itself. Once doubts have been sown about potential vaccine risks – even where these have proved to be unsubstantiated – public health officials have found it difficult to convince an increasingly distrustful public of the extremely high safety record of vaccines. Moreover, the global reach of the Internet has ensured that unsubstantiated information on reactions to immunization can travel much more quickly and reach a wider audience. The fears of a distrusting public in the developed countries may be quickly repeated as 'facts', negatively affecting coverage in the developing countries, where failure to immunize often has disastrous consequences.

In the less-developed countries unsafe injection practices are rife and account for an estimated US$ 535 million a year in health care costs and 1.3 million deaths a year

Injection safety

Lives are also put at risk in many developing countries by failure to ensure injection safety. While in the developed countries problems are largely restricted to injecting drug use and occasional needle-stick injuries among health workers, in the less-developed countries unsafe injection practices are rife and account for an estimated US$ 535 million a year in health care costs and 1.3 million deaths a year.

However, injections for immunization account for less than 10% of all injections for medical purposes and are generally considered to be safer than curative injections, which include many unnecessary and unsafe injections.

Since the 1980s, WHO, UNICEF and other partners, have provided training on injection safety, and over the past decade have advocated the introduction of single-use autodisable (AD) syringes, which have a blocking mechanism to prevent their re-use. However, the practice of re-using unsterile needles and syringes has continued in some countries.

** An AEFI is the term used to describe a medical incident that is associated with the vaccine used, but may not necessarily be associated causally with the vaccine. In reality, most of these incidents are not vaccine-related.*

A 1998 study involving 19 countries in five regions in the developing world found that in 14 countries at least 50% of injections were unsafe. Overall, unsafe injection practices in developing countries were identified as the cause of at least 8 million hepatitis B infections a year, 2 million hepatitis C infections, and 75 000 cases of HIV/AIDS, as well as cases of Ebola, Lassa fever, dengue and malaria. Other estimates suggested the number of infections could be twice as high.

In 1994, a conference in Côte d'Ivoire involving more than 50 African countries endorsed the Yamoussoukro Declaration, which set a target of 95% safe injections by 1997. But that target is far from being met in many developing countries today. A study on safety of immunization injections in 13 African countries carried out between 1995 and 1998, concluded that there had been no progress on injection safety in these countries over the previous decade.

This study revealed that injection equipment was being re-used without sterilization, a substantial proportion of health centres had a shortage of injection equipment, and used syringes and needles were found both in and around the health centres. In some countries, unqualified staff were in charge of sterilization procedures, sterilization equipment was not working properly due to a lack of spare parts or fuel shortages, and quality assurance functions did not exist.

As the use of single-use AD syringes has increased in developing countries, so too has the volume of hazardous waste that needs to be buried or incinerated. The inadequate disposal of medical waste, including contaminated needles and syringes, creates an additional health hazard, particularly in low-income countries. Even where countries have adequate disposal facilities, the transport and storage of medical waste can expose both children and adults to contaminated needles and syringes. In poor countries culturally opposed to waste, the commercial incentive to scavenge and recycle even hazardous medical waste may be irresistible.

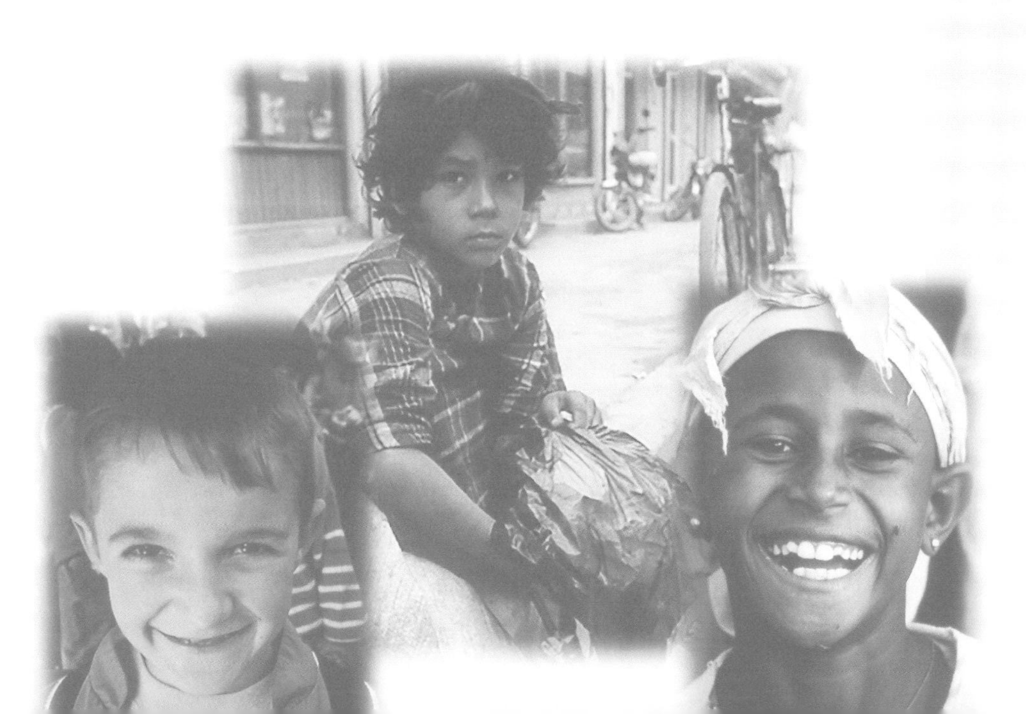

6. Finance gaps

This section highlights the failure of both national governments and international donors over the past decade to invest sufficiently in immunization programmes in developing countries.

Developing countries account for 93% of the world's disease burden but only 18% of its income and only 11% of global spending on health

Routine immunization programmes have been neglected as funding has failed to keep up with population growth and the higher cost of delivering services. In some cases, absolute funding levels have fallen dramatically due to withdrawal of donor support and greater pressure on public spending.

Furthermore, some of the poorest, most heavily indebted countries are spending three to five times as much on debt repayments as on basic services for their people. Health economists at the World Bank estimate that developing countries account for 93% of the world's disease burden but only 18% of its income and only 11% of global spending on health.

Figure 5: **Cost profile of immunization programmes***
Range of cost per fully immunized child

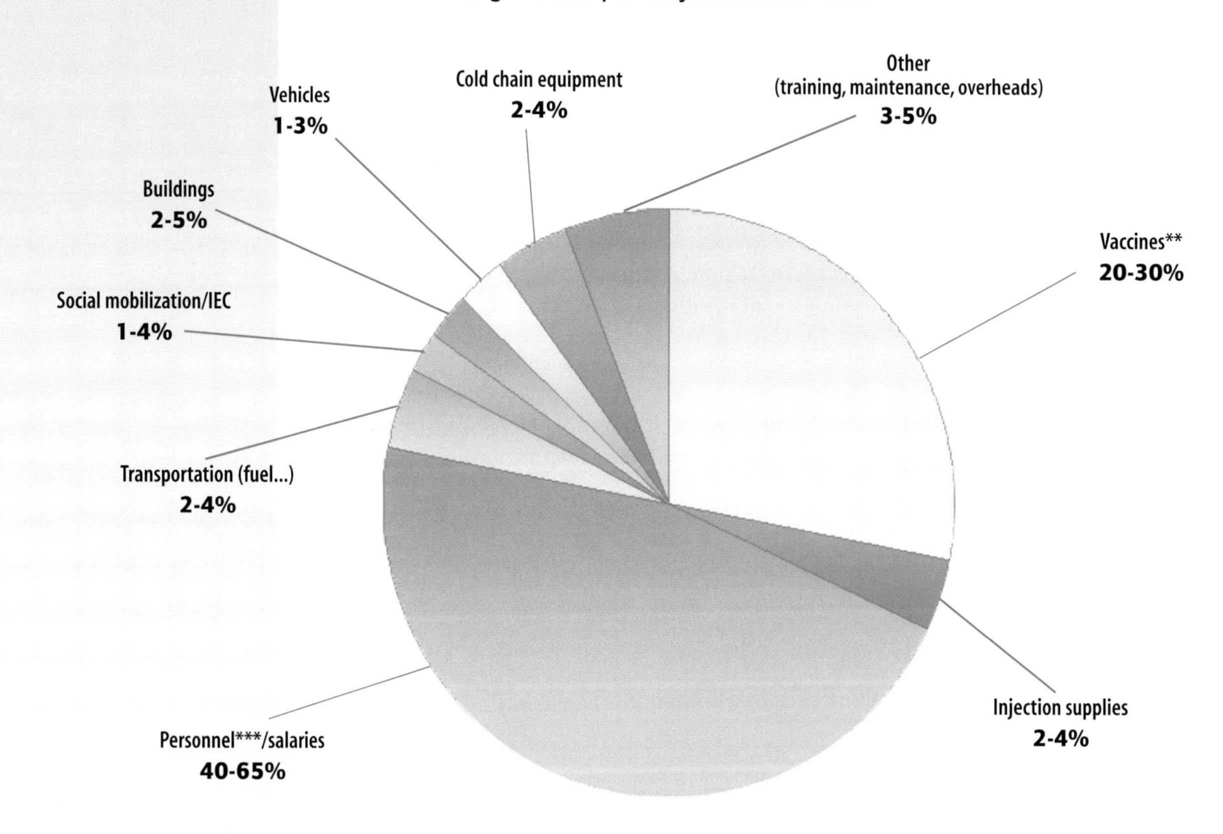

* *Based on a selection of in-depth developing country-specific costing studies.*
** *The share of vaccines will vary depending on different country vaccination schedules and will be greater with the introduction of new vaccines.*
*** *Personnel costs are likely to be the main cost driver of immunization programmes. These costs will vary across countries depending on differences In wage levels and whether shared personnel costs are included.*

Source: GAVI Financing Task Force

Unpredictable funding can also greatly reduce the effectiveness of immunization programmes. The health benefits of immunization depend on reaching high levels of coverage among generation after generation of children – an achievement that can ultimately interrupt the transmission of some diseases. However, a sudden lack of funding and a shortage of personnel, vaccines or cold chain fuel can lead to a breakdown in the immunization system and to outbreaks of disease that can put millions of lives at risk (see Fig. 5).

Immunization is one of the state's core public health responsibilities in both developed and developing countries. However, many governments in low-income countries do not allocate adequate and reliable financial resources to immunization. Even with donor support, the least-developed countries spend on average only US$ 6 per capita a year on all health services, including immunization. But the 2001 report of the WHO-sponsored Commission on Macroeconomics and Health declared that far more, at least US$ 30–40 per capita, was needed to ensure a package of essential interventions to meet the basic health needs of the population.

Commission on Macroeconomics and Health

The key recommendation of the Commission is that the world's low- and middle-income countries, should scale up the access of the world's poor to essential health services, including a focus on specific interventions

Immunization may be even more disadvantaged than other health services in the allocation of government funds. In common with other preventive services, immunization has no organized constituency and often loses out when competing with high profile curative services for scarce resources. In addition, the priority-setting of donor agencies has inadvertently contributed to the relatively low level of government spending on immunization in some low-income countries. Over the years, many donor agencies have focused their support on maternal and child health programmes, including immunization. However, the willingness of the international community to pay for vaccines and other inputs has enabled the government to divert scarce resources to other pressing demands in some countries. Immunization programmes suffer from funding uncertainties, competition from both within and outside the health sector, and increases in funding requirements as coverage expands and new vaccines become available. This occurs even in developing countries with a relatively higher national income. Overall, developing countries are getting further from achieving the benefits of immunization as realized in developed countries, and the rich-poor immunization gap will continue to grow if left to domestic government resources alone. END Part 1

Part 2: Charting a way forward

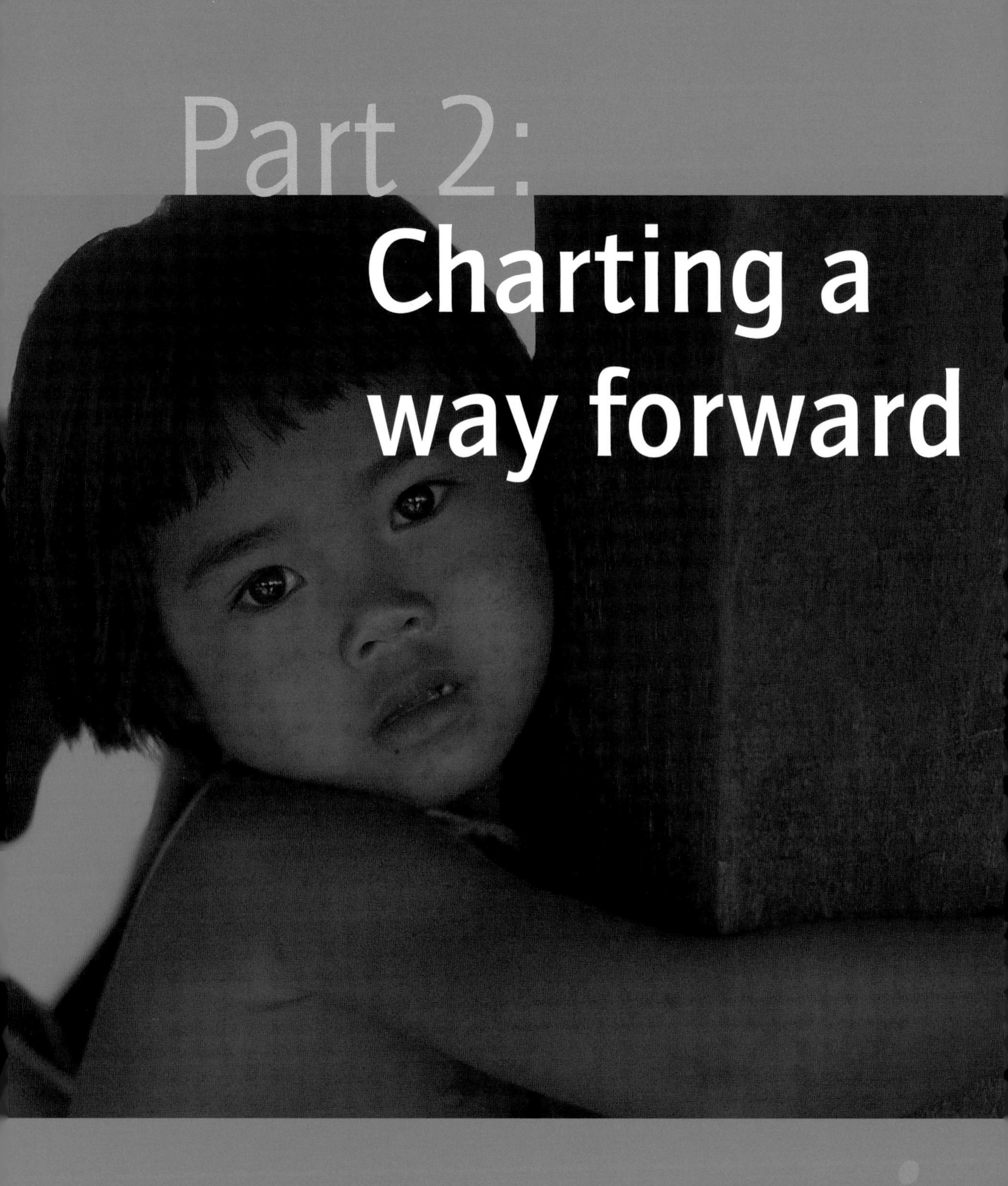

Part 2 of this report looks at what is currently being done and what more needs to be done to re-energize and strengthen immunization services in developing countries and close the gaps in access to vaccines and immunization. It outlines the GAVI approach; new strategies to speed up the research, development and introduction of priority new vaccines for poor countries; efforts to improve immunization systems (including immunization safety); and the search for new and improved sustainable financing mechanisms for immunization.

Among the new approaches highlighted in this section are:

- The use of performance-related funding to boost immunization coverage
- More pragmatic working relationships between the public sector and the vaccine industry to ensure the R&D of vaccines for use in developing countries
- New measures to improve immunization systems (including immunization safety)
- Innovative ways of reaching the most difficult-to-reach populations
- The use of immunization as a gateway for other low-cost health interventions
- New funding mechanisms.

's save lives

1. The power of partnership: GAVI

This section looks at the efforts by GAVI partners to boost immunization coverage and improve access to under-used vaccines in developing countries.

In response to mounting international concern at low immunization coverage, the growing inequalities in immunization and the unacceptable toll of infectious diseases in developing countries, new global partnerships have been forged to break the cycle of neglect. Foremost among these is the Global Alliance for Vaccines and Immunization (GAVI), which brings together major stakeholders in immunization from both the public and private sector. These stakeholders include WHO, UNICEF, the World Bank Group, national governments, international development banks, bilateral agencies, nongovernmental organizations (NGOs), the Bill & Melinda Gates Foundation, the Children's Vaccine Program at the Program for Appropriate Technology for Health (PATH), foundations, public health programmes, and representatives of the vaccine industry from both developing and developed countries. Together, these partners offer a range of skills in the fields of vaccine research, production, supply, immunization programme delivery, international financing mechanisms, and advocacy and communications.

Global Alliance for Vaccines and Immunization (GAVI)

Launched in early 2000, the Alliance is designed to:

- Realize the right of every child to immunization against the major infectious diseases
- Improve immunization systems (including immunization safety) in developing countries
- Increase coverage with new and existing vaccines
- Accelerate the R&D of priority vaccines for use mainly in developing countries
- Develop new sustainable funding mechanisms for immunization in the poorest countries
- Promote tiered pricing so as to lower the price of new vaccines for the poorest countries
- Use immunization as a platform for the delivery of other cost-effective health interventions
- Develop new ways of reaching the most-difficult-to-reach children who currently slip through the net
- Promote the development and use of new simpler and safer vaccine technologies and delivery systems to increase coverage and improve immunization safety
- Establish immunization as one of the key performance indicators to measure the success of international development efforts, including debt relief initiatives.
- Support national and international accelerated disease control targets for vaccine preventable diseases.

The Alliance operates through a new financing mechanism, the Vaccine Fund, established with an initial grant of US$ 750 million over five years from the Bill & Melinda Gates Foundation, which has been boosted to US$ 1 billion by contributions from the governments of Canada, Denmark, the Netherlands, Norway, Sweden, the United Kingdom, the United States and private contributors. The goal is to raise US$ 2 billion over five years.

New ways of working

Since 2000, the GAVI partners have been targeting assistance to the poorest countries through the Vaccine Fund to help them boost coverage with existing vaccines, improve immunization systems (including injection safety) and introduce under-used vaccines, including hepatitis B, Hib and yellow fever. To qualify for support from the Vaccine Fund, countries must have a per capita GNP of not more than US$ 1000 and immunization coverage (with DTP) below 80%. Progress so far has been dramatic.

Over 70 of the poorest countries are eligible for support from the Vaccine Fund. Within two years, 90% of these countries had applied for assistance. The Vaccine Fund has awarded over US$ 800 million in grants over five years to 54 countries including war-torn countries such as Afghanistan, Liberia and Sierra Leone, and three populous countries: China, India and Indonesia. In addition to the substantial national and international financing of immunization programmes, GAVI partners estimate this investment will help increase basic immunization rates in funded countries by 17% and boost coverage with hepatitis B vaccine from 18% to 65% by 2007, potentially preventing over 2 million deaths.

Countries apply for funding by sending proposals to the GAVI Secretariat, outlining a three to five-year plan designed to boost immunization coverage. The plan must be based on a recent comprehensive assessment of the immunization programme and endorsed by the national interagency coordinating committee (ICC).

These committees – typically chaired by the Ministry of Health and with representation from agencies such as WHO, UNICEF, bilateral agencies and NGOs – sustain the progress of the work-plans as well as galvanizing and coordinating partner support (see Box).

The GAVI Board reviews the proposals and makes recommendations to the Vaccine Fund for the disbursement of funds. Countries with low levels of immunization coverage (under 50% fully immunized with DTP) can obtain grant funding for five years to help improve their immunization services and increase coverage with the traditional childhood vaccines. What is novel about this approach is that the funds are not earmarked. Governments and interagency coordinating committees jointly decide how best to use the funds, e.g. it could be spent on re-equipping the cold chain, on training additional health workers, or even just increasing the district budget to support local priorities.

The GAVI funding is based on the innovative idea of a "share" of US$ 20 for every additional child which the government commits to immunize. Half of this amount is paid upfront and the rest as a reward for each child actually immunized, subject to an independent audit. Once a country has increased immunization coverage to at least 50% they can apply for an additional grant for the introduction of new vaccines. However, continued support for immunization services will depend on the government achieving its targets (the number of children immunized, for example), and these must be validated by transparent monitoring systems.

Interagency coordinating committees (ICCs)

ICCs are a key coordinating mechanism for immunization services in developing countries. First established in the Americas to support the polio eradication initiative, their mandate has recently been extended to include all aspects of immunization.

The ICCs operate under the aegis of the national government. Membership includes government ministries, major partner agencies (WHO, UNICEF and bilateral agencies), nongovernmental organizations and the private sector. In some countries, similar committees have been established to coordinate issues relating to the broader health sector.

The ICCs have wide-ranging responsibility for issues relating to immunization including:

- **technical support** (developing national immunization policy and strategic plans of action, monitoring programme performance and quality control mechanisms)
- **financial support** (mobilizing resources and monitoring the appropriate use of available resources)
- **political support** (social mobilization and advocacy to help increase political commitment for immunization)
- **capacity building** (to ensure government ownership of the administration and delivery of national immunization programmes).

Countries with moderate levels of coverage with the basic EPI vaccines (50–80% coverage with DTP) are also eligible for five years of grant funding for the introduction of new and under-used vaccines against hepatitis B and Hib (where appropriate), including the cost of safe injection equipment. However, yellow fever vaccine is being made available to countries, where needed, regardless of their DTP status. All governments receiving Vaccine Fund support for new vaccines are expected to prepare financial sustainability plans outlining the actions they will take to mobilize sustainable resources – both from their own budget and from external sources – well before the funding period comes to an end.

Achieving the common targets

The GAVI partners have committed to achieve ambitious targets aimed at increasing access to immunization, introducing under-used vaccines (hepatitis B, Hib and yellow fever), and accelerating the development and introduction of new vaccines such as pneumococcal, rotavirus and meningitis (see Fig. 6).

Inevitably there have been a few teething problems, with complaints that the initial application process was too fast and time-consuming for countries and that the fixed share price of US$ 20 per child immunized is unfair because it discriminates against countries with hard-to-reach populations such as Chad and Niger – where it costs far more to immunize a child, especially in remote rural areas.

In addition, the focus on assisting countries with weak health service delivery systems led to increased demand for combination vaccines, which protect children against several diseases in a single shot. As a result, demand outstripped supply and a temporary shortage of these vaccines occurred. However, manufacturers are already taking steps to increase production capacity to meet the demand for combination vaccines. In the meantime, supplies of hepatitis B vaccine in monovalent form remain available.

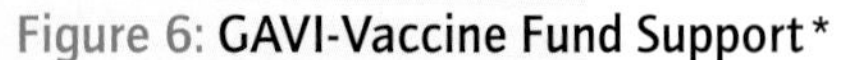
Figure 6: GAVI-Vaccine Fund Support*

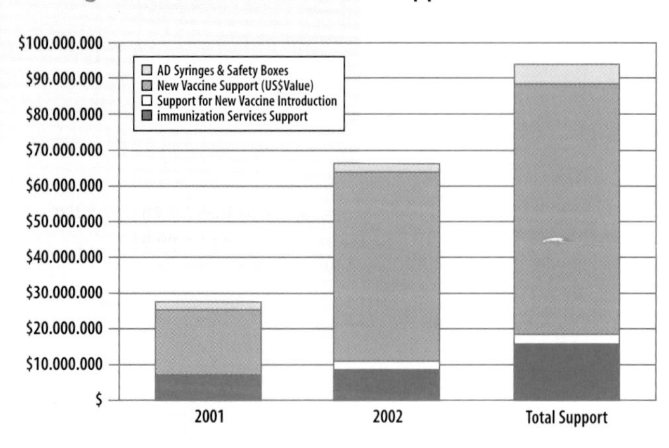

Source: GAVI Financing Task Force
**Actual disbursements*

Another challenge is the performance-based grants system, which rewards countries for the additional number of children immunized. Its implementation has had to be postponed to give countries more time to improve their reporting systems and ensure that their immunization data can be audited and verified. As a result, countries will continue to receive increased investment support before being assessed for their reward payment a year later than envisaged at the outset.

In the meantime, it is anticipated that the new commitment to finance existing under-used vaccines will now spur the vaccine industry to invest in the R&D of priority new vaccines for developing countries.

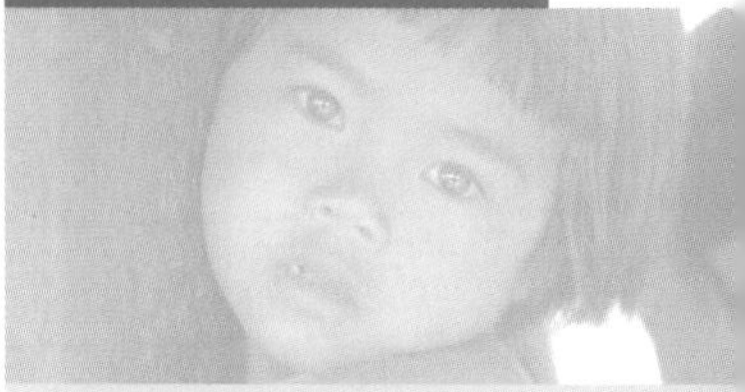

2. Development and introduction of new vaccines

This section highlights recent trends in the vaccine market and outlines new initiatives to ensure the research and development of priority vaccines for developing countries. It emphasizes the need to establish developing country demand in addition to a commitment to buy a new vaccine at an earlier stage in the vaccine cycle in order to guarantee both adequate supplies and lower prices.

Guaranteeing a market

While the market for vaccines in developing countries is potentially vast – including the 132 million children born each year – they currently account for only 18% of the global US$ 6 billion vaccine market. Their uptake of newer, more expensive vaccines has been slow and uncertain in recent years – leading to doubts about the public sector's ability to forecast demand, backed up by the necessary resources. To further complicate matters, demand for vaccines has been erratic. Efforts to provide accurate forecasts of demand have been hampered by one-year funding cycles, when lead times for vaccine production can be as long as three to five years. As a result, until recently, the developing country market was perceived to be risky and relatively small.

For manufacturers to ensure an adequate and regular supply of vaccines, a forecast of demand, backed by sustainable financing, is needed several years in advance. The public sector needs to do far more to estimate the burden of disease, forecast demand and guarantee a market for new vaccines in developing countries. A firm commitment upfront to purchase safe and effective vaccines will reduce the risks faced by private sector manufacturers and help re-direct global research towards the vaccines that are a priority for developing countries. In addition, predictable market conditions can help secure the availability and affordability of new vaccines – through credible demand forecasts, bulk purchasing schemes and futures agreements. Figure 7 outlines the immunization cycle from vaccine research to disease prevention, highlighting the critical importance of ensuring vaccine production, supply and finance.

Figure 7: **Immunization – from research to disease prevention**

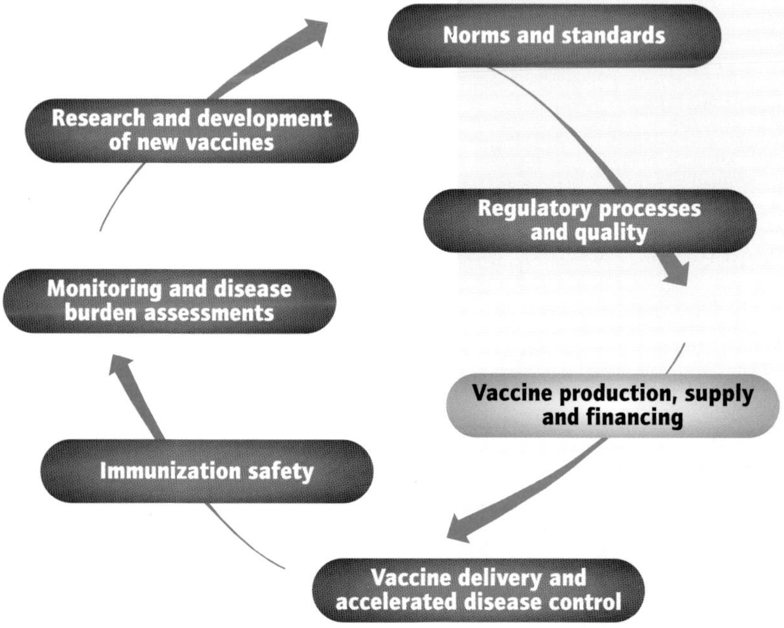

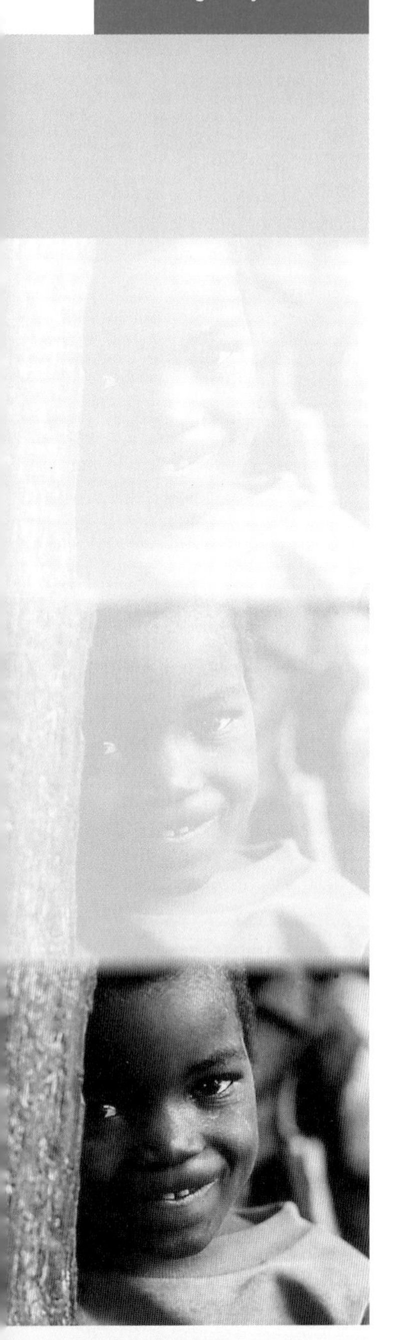

A recent study carried out for the GAVI partners proposed a new strategy for the accelerated development and introduction of two priority vaccines for developing countries, a pneumococcal congugate vaccine and a rotavirus vaccine. The accelerated development and introduction plans (ADIPs) involve efforts to help countries establish credible forecasts of vaccine demand (based on the disease burden and the safety and efficacy of the vaccine) at an early stage in the vaccine cycle, i.e. before manufacturers undertake the lengthy development and scale-up process. By removing this uncertainty, manufacturers will be better able to meet global supply needs and the increased production volume should help lower prices. Meanwhile, early forecasts of demand will enable developing countries to secure sustainable financing from national sources and to negotiate additional funding from donors to fill the gaps. It has been estimated that the new strategy could advance the introduction of these vaccines in developing countries by six years, preventing an estimated 2.2 million deaths from streptococcus pneumonia and 1.1 million deaths from rotavirus by 2020.

One way of offsetting some of the costs of vaccine R&D is the use of innovative funding support mechanisms such as the Vaccine Fund and the Global Fund to Fight AIDS, Tuberculosis and Malaria. These organizations can also help lobby for low vaccine prices and act as a catalyst for research by providing a credible market for new and existing products. Funds are to be made available through the Vaccine Fund, for example, to help accelerate the development of vaccines for use in the least-developed countries against pneumococcal disease, rotavirus and meningitis.

Another way of guaranteeing a future market as an incentive for R&D is the use of loans or a purchase fund whose use is contingent on the successful development of a vaccine. Financing – to cover the full price of the vaccine or a per dose subsidy in addition to government spending – would be available only for a product that met certain pre-determined criteria (such as efficacy, cost effectiveness and reasonable price), thereby providing both an incentive and a means of regulating the market.

Tax breaks can also be used to give manufacturers incentives to accelerate R&D for vaccines against diseases of poverty. The UK government has announced plans for a tax credit payable to UK-registered pharmaceutical companies for the development of vaccines or drugs for HIV/AIDS, tuberculosis and malaria. Tax deductions will also be used to encourage industry donations of medical supplies (including drugs and vaccines) and equipment to support developing country strategies to combat diseases of poverty. Also, in the United States, legislation is pending on plans to introduce tax credits for R&D for vaccines against HIV/AIDS, tuberculosis, malaria and any other diseases that account for over one million deaths a year.

Clinical trials

Efforts are also needed to strengthen the capacity of developing countries to carry out trials of priority vaccines for use among the poorest populations. Only a limited number of research centres exist with the capacity and experience needed to conduct large-scale clinical trials of new vaccines, which can involve tens of thousands of people over several years. As a result, progress is stalled on some of the vaccines already being developed which are urgently needed in developing countries. In order to solve this dilemma, the public sector needs to work in partnership with vaccine manufacturers to build the capacity needed in developing countries for applied vaccine research, clinical evaluation and early introduction of priority new vaccines. Public-private vaccine partnerships, such as the Malaria Vaccine Initiative (MVI) and the IAVI, are already funding a number of clinical trials in developing country settings.

Parallel clinical trials are essential to evaluate key differences in the use of a vaccine among populations in developing and developed countries. These include variations in the serotype or strain of the disease-causing organism, the effectiveness of the vaccine among different populations and possible variations in the required dosage. Until recently, vaccines were often already licensed or at a very advanced stage of development before they were tested in developing countries. Today, it is recognized that clinical trials – and burden of disease studies – must be carried out in developing countries at an early stage in order to establish accurate forecasts of demand and speed up access to new vaccines at affordable prices. In turn, this will spur vaccine manufacturers to continue to invest in vaccine R&D for developing countries.

Tiered pricing

Once a new vaccine has been licensed for use, tiered pricing is a way of avoiding the 10–20 year delay in access to new vaccines for the poorest countries. The premise of tiered pricing is that new vaccines for use in developing countries would be made available at reduced prices – the lower price being offset by the higher prices paid for the same product in richer markets. In this way, manufacturers would be able to recoup their investments and make the product available to developing country markets at the same time.

Vaccine prices are already tiered in most cases, with prices tailored to different markets. UNICEF, for example, buys vaccines in bulk for use in the poorest countries and negotiates lower prices than those paid for the same product in the developed countries. In 2000, UNICEF purchased over 2.4 billion doses of vaccine worth US$ 151 million, including almost 2 billion doses of OPV.

The success of tiered pricing has only been possible because of the support of developed countries and the willingness of their governments and public to pay more than developing countries for vaccines. Many believe that achieving the GAVI partners' ambitious targets will require price tiering at an earlier stage in the product cycle as well as differentiated prices for low-, middle- and high-income countries.

Another low-cost source of vaccines is the revolving fund established by the Pan American Health Organization (PAHO) in the late 1970s. The fund pools vaccine orders for countries in Latin America, buys vaccine at reduced prices, and

While new vaccine development is today carried out mainly by large multinational manufacturers, developing country manufacturers are already playing a major role in manufacturing and in the future they are expected to play an increasing role in product development

supplies vaccine to countries at a standard, stable price. The concession is conditional on the introduction of a separate item for immunization in the national health budget, development of a five-year immunization plan, and oversight by a national immunization programme manager. It also has the capacity to function as an emergency fund, swiftly re-routing supplies in the event of an outbreak of disease. The fund currently has a purchasing power of approximately US$ 145 million.

Recent trends in the vaccine market

Over the past decade, a series of mergers between some of the major pharmaceutical companies, coupled with the shrinking manufacturing base for low-profit traditional vaccines, has resulted in a global shortage of some vaccines. The reduction in the number of suppliers to the global market has made vaccine supply vulnerable to lot failures, further contributing to recent vaccine shortages (see Fig. 8).

While new vaccine development is today carried out mainly by large multinational manufacturers, developing country manufacturers are already playing a major role in manufacturing and in the future they are expected to play an increasing role in product development. For example, even after excluding polio vaccine, 50% of UNICEF's vaccine procurement in 2000 was purchased from these so-called "emerging producers". Although many are still building R&D capacity, they already have a major influence on the global supply picture. Ultimately, the manufacture of an adequate supply of safe, effective vaccines by multinationals and developing country manufacturers will help ensure a sustainable supply of vaccine as well as a faster reduction in price.

Several developing country manufacturers have entered into joint agreements with major vaccine manufacturers for the production of some vaccines. They include Biomanguinhos (Brazil) with GlaxoSmithKline for Hib vaccine, the Instituto Butantán (Brazil) with Aventis Pasteur for influenza vaccine, the Instituto Finlay (Cuba) with Glaxo SmithKline for meningococcal group B vaccine, and VacSera (Egypt) with GlaxoSmithKline for the DTP-HepB combination. In addition, the Cuba-based Centre for Genetic Engineering and Biotechnology (CIGB) has successfully transferred its technology to another developing country vaccine manufacturer, and is currently executing other technology transfers and negotiating new agreements.

In 2000, several high quality vaccine manufacturers established a developing country vaccine manufacturers network. The manufacturers are working together to develop innovative strategies for the production of the high-quality vaccines needed. One initiative involves negotiations to combine the

Figure 8: Manufacturers leaving the developing country market, 1992-2001

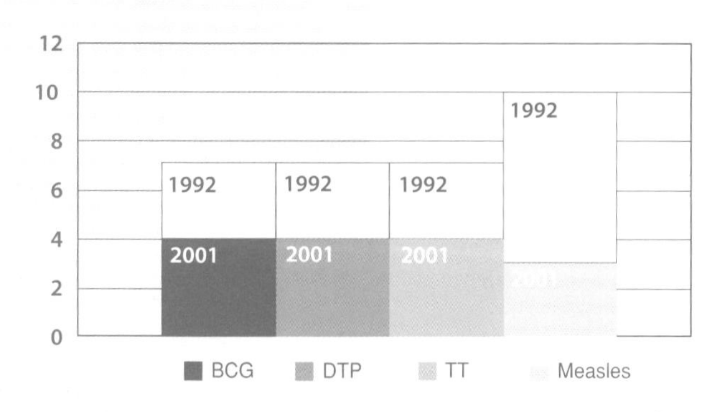

Source: GAVI Secretariat

various pre-qualified vaccines – such as diphtheria, tetanus, and whole cell pertussis (DTwP), hepatitis B and Hib – into various combinations for use in developing countries. These are expected to be available by 2005.

Another recent phenomenon is the increasing divergence between vaccine schedules in high-income and low- and middle-income countries, which may have an impact on both the supply and price of vaccines for use in developing countries. The problem is two-fold: first, the introduction of new vaccines to meet the needs of developed countries (such as pneumococcal and meningoccocal conjugate vaccines, based on the forms of the bacteria that circulate in developed countries); and secondly, the development of new vaccine substitutions to meet the increased regulatory requirements of the developed countries. These include acellular pertussis vaccine to replace the whole cell pertussis component of DTP vaccine, and Inactivated Polio Vaccine (IPV) to replace live Oral Polio Vaccine (OPV), while whole cell pertussis and OPV are still used in developing countries. In addition, the removal of the mercury-based preservative thiomersal from vaccines in response to recommendations from regulatory bodies in the developed countries, has resulted in a switch to more expensive single-dose vaccine vials for developed country markets and placed greater demands on manufacturing capacity, thereby increasing the fragility of the vaccine supply chain (see Box on thiomersal p. 32). Meanwhile, the divergence in vaccine schedules and the lack of excess production capacity could potentially undermine the practice of tiered pricing in which low-income countries obtain vaccine at a lower price offset by the higher price paid for the same product in developed countries.

3. Improving immunization services

This section highlights efforts to strengthen immunization services and health service delivery systems in developing countries. It looks at the role of immunization in providing a platform for other essential health services and outlines new strategies to identify and target the hard-to-reach children who miss out on immunization. This section also underlines the importance of harnessing new technology to boost immunization coverage and safety and outlines a range of new initiatives to assure the quality and safety of vaccines and to improve injection safety.

Capacity building support

In each country, immunization services exist within the wider context of the overall health system. Immunization is likely to suffer in countries where health service infrastructure is poor and delivery systems are under-resourced and poorly managed. However, immunization services can also assist in improving health systems, e.g. through establishing best practices and providing opportunities for the delivery of other cost-effective health interventions. This has been illustrated by the polio eradication initiative – the largest ever public health initiative –

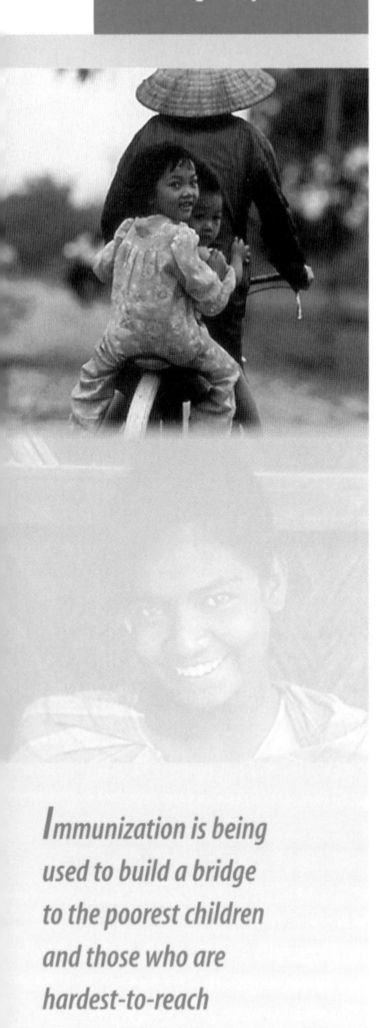

Immunization is being used to build a bridge to the poorest children and those who are hardest-to-reach

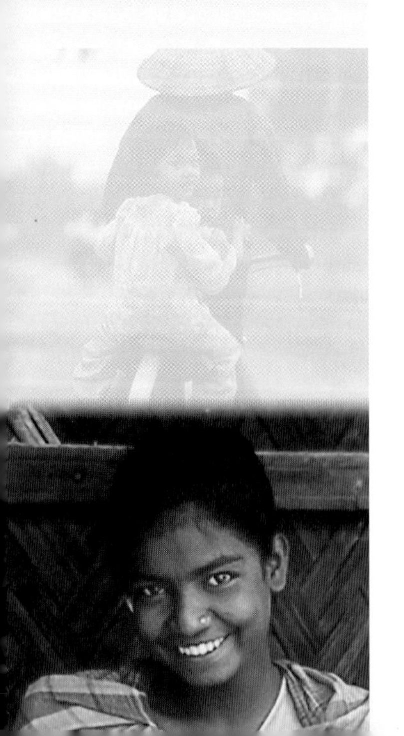

which has led the way in strengthening national surveillance systems, improving cold chain systems and establishing a global laboratory network that is already being used for other disease control activities. This initiative has also demonstrated that it is possible to reach children even in the remotest areas or in countries affected by war. Innovative methods such as house-to-house (even boat-to-boat) visits, large-scale social mobilization, and even brokering "Days of Tranquillity" where weapons are laid aside for national immunization days, have all been introduced in seeking to eradicate polio. This has shown what can be achieved with wide-ranging support from national and international NGOs and other partners, and the mobilization of a global force of millions of volunteers. Today, efforts are under way not only to ensure sustainable funding for immunization programmes but also to strengthen managerial capacity at both national and district level, improve immunization safety, increase immunization coverage by targeting the unreached, and use systems more effectively so as to introduce new vaccines. The challenge for these countries is to mobilize national budgets that can be complemented by external support.

Countries that apply for funding support through GAVI may be eligible to receive funding both for vaccines and capacity building support. This support is contingent on countries carrying out an overall assessment of their immunization services, using a set of agreed standards to identify their current strengths and weaknesses. On the basis of this, countries are establishing a multi-year plan of action for immunization in addition to making commitments to meet targets for raising coverage and strengthening any weak links in the system. In addition, national governments and development partners are being urged to ensure that immunization services are central to health sector development plans and that immunization targets are used as key performance indicators for development.

In many developing countries, health system reform, often involving the decentralization of health services and a shift from tertiary to primary health care, has brought services closer to the people who use them, thereby providing opportunities for more effective targeting of services and greater responsiveness to local needs. Provided that certain key immunization functions – such as vaccine procurement – remain at the central level, health sector reform can offer opportunities to improve the performance of immunization services by boosting the performance of district-level disease monitoring and reporting systems, for example, and ensuring better targeting of poor and under-served populations.

In Ghana, for example, which adopted a Sector Wide Approach (SWAP) to health system reform based on an agreed package of social service reforms and financed by the pooling of donor funds, immunization was established as one of the key performance indicators for resource allocation. In order to both increase coverage and meet targets, private health care workers (including midwives) were employed to boost staffing levels so as to enable the expansion of outreach services. As a result, immunization coverage increased by about 20% between 1997 and 1998.

Immunization as a platform for other health services

In countries where there is no recognizable health infrastructure, or where health services barely exist outside urban areas, immunization is being used to build a bridge to the poorest children and those who are hardest-to-reach. In 1999, for example, in the war-torn Democratic Republic of Congo, the first nationwide polio immunization campaigns brought health care to some children for the very first time. While the use of immunization campaigns to deliver other health services is especially important for children who have no regular contact with health services, routine immunization services can also be the platform for a range of other cost-effective health interventions, such as micronutrient supplements and routine health checks.

Supplements of vitamin A taken every four to six months can reduce child mortality from all causes by as much as 23%, measles mortality by 50% and diarrhoeal disease mortality by 33%. The challenge facing health planners is how to devise a viable and low-cost delivery mechanism to provide vitamin A supplements to the estimated 250 million children at risk. One of the quickest and most successful strategies has been to link vitamin A delivery with polio and measles vaccination campaigns. In 2000, over 60 countries delivered vitamin A during national immunization days. Many countries have already linked vitamin A delivery with routine immunization services. The long-term aim is to ensure that vitamin A is integrated into all routine immunization programmes.

Supplements of vitamin A taken every four to six months can reduce child mortality from all causes by as much as 23%, measles mortality by 50% and diarrhoeal disease mortality by 33%

Elsewhere, a research study in Tanzania involving 700 children has used routine immunization visits to deliver preventive treatment for malaria and anaemia, major causes of hospital admission and mortality among children in developing countries. During the first year of life, this treatment reduced the incidence of clinical malaria by almost 60%, the incidence of severe anaemia by 50% and the rate of hospital admission by 30% when compared with children in the control group who were not treated. If these preliminary findings are confirmed by follow-up studies, this treatment would be possible to deliver both with conventional routine strategies and through sustained outreach strategies.

Reaching the unreached

In an effort to identify and target the children who slip through the net and remain unvaccinated, countries are increasingly introducing district-level monitoring and performance targets. This gives a truer picture of immunization coverage than national averages which can conceal huge disparities between rich and poor. Within Ethiopia, for example, coverage can vary from below 10% to 80%, because of the difficulty in reaching nomadic populations.

Of the one in four children who miss out on immunization every year, many live in remote areas beyond the reach of health services. Specialized strategies are needed to reach these populations, including some who are nomadic and therefore even more difficult to reach. But efforts to vaccinate these children will be expensive – about five times more than what it costs to immunize children in a densely populated urban area.

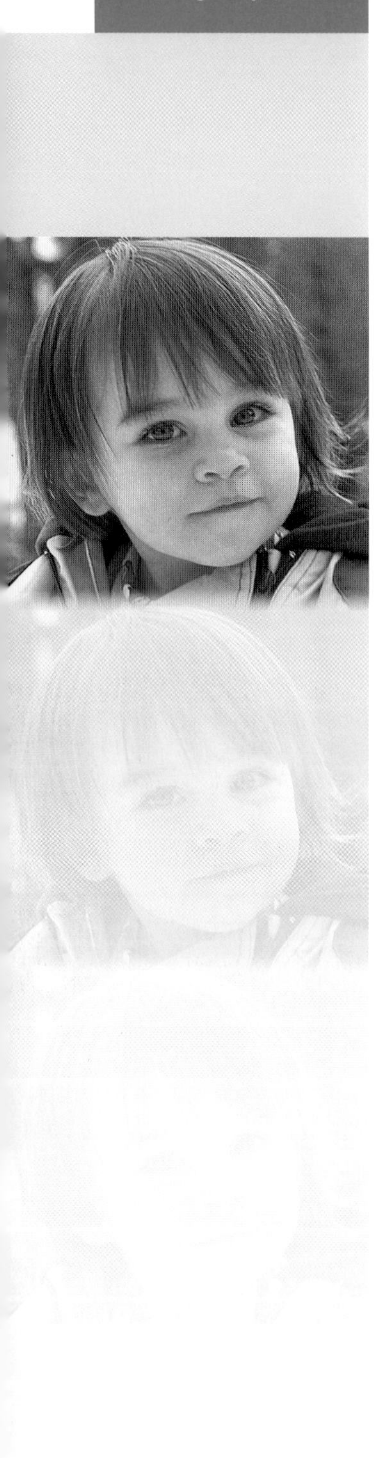

Another challenge is to reach the unreached in urban areas where immunization coverage is sometimes lower than in rural areas. The problem is that basic health services in cities are all too often stretched beyond their capacity by the vast number of people they are expected to serve. Among those who slip through the net are the children of migrant workers who are regularly on the move and have no extended family to support them when government services fail.

The development of Sustainable Outreach Services (SOS) is an innovative way of providing a minimum package of essential services, tailored to local needs, for populations living in remote areas. Uptake of services is dependent on effective social mobilization efforts – to establish a demand for immunization, for example, and ensure community ownership of the overall scheme. Basic health services on offer include immunization, vitamin A and other micronutrient supplementation, malaria control (including distribution of bednets), traditional birth attendant training and supply of safe delivery kits, family planning and anti-parasitic treatments. Where the community identifies a need, health services can be used as a springboard for other services such as agricultural advice, cattle immunization, decontamination of wells and latrine construction. The community negotiates the kind of service needed and supervises its delivery.

Contact may then be made from one to three times a year, over several days – a strategy that can be just as effective and far more efficient than using a fixed site. SOS share many of the aspects of routine delivery, but a higher degree of flexibility is needed in view of the difficult terrain and the unpredictability of delivery. Efficient transport management systems are critical in efforts to reach remote populations, with forms of transport ranging from four-wheel drive vehicles, motorcycles and bicycles, to camels and boats.

SOS build on the successful relationship with nongovernmental organizations working in immunization. In Mozambique, for example, Save the Children Fund supports a sustained outreach strategy, through a joint agreement with UNICEF and the Provincial Directorate of Health. Immunization and other health services are now being made available to 430 000 people in two districts with low immunization coverage. Elsewhere, in a remote area of Uganda, the British NGO Riders for Health helps purchase motorcycles and manage a maintenance service to ensure the delivery of outreach services to 400 000 people. Health services available include immunization for children and pregnant mothers, oral rehydration and family planning. Meanwhile, in Cambodia, a network of 15 NGOs is supporting a health outreach programme targeting over 1000 remote villages in forested areas; in this example, the distribution of bednets is being used as a platform for other cost-effective health interventions including malaria treatment, immunization, vitamin A, leprosy screening and de-worming treatments.

Harnessing new technology

New improved vaccine technologies and delivery systems can also be used to increase immunization coverage by reducing the number of contacts needed, lowering delivery costs and enabling vaccine to be used beyond the cold chain. The use of the vaccine vial monitor (VVM), for example – an ingenious heat-sensitive label on a vaccine vial – is revolutionizing the way vaccines are delivered, bringing vaccine to greater numbers of children in remote areas and cutting down on vaccine waste. This invention takes the guesswork out of knowing whether vaccine has been damaged by heat exposure during transport or storage. In southern Sudan and Somalia, for example, VVMs have shown that vaccine could still be used after long journeys to remote areas in temperatures of up to 40° Celsius.

Before the device was introduced in 1996 – initially on polio vaccine vials – health workers were trained to exercise necessary caution and throw vaccine away after any suspected break in the cold chain. VVMs have now cut vaccine wastage by up to 45% in some countries.

Another breakthrough that may greatly improve vaccine delivery in remote areas is the development of the Uniject™, a prefilled injection device that is already being used in Mali as part of global efforts to eliminate maternal and neonatal tetanus. Uniject™ is an AD syringe combined with a single dose of vaccine that can be used more safely, easily and accurately by community vaccinators. When filled with a heat-stable vaccine such as TT or hepatitis B vaccine, it can readily be stored outside the cold chain and used to reach people in the remotest communities. The device was developed by PATH, with support from USAID, in order to prevent the re-use of needles and to simplify immunization.

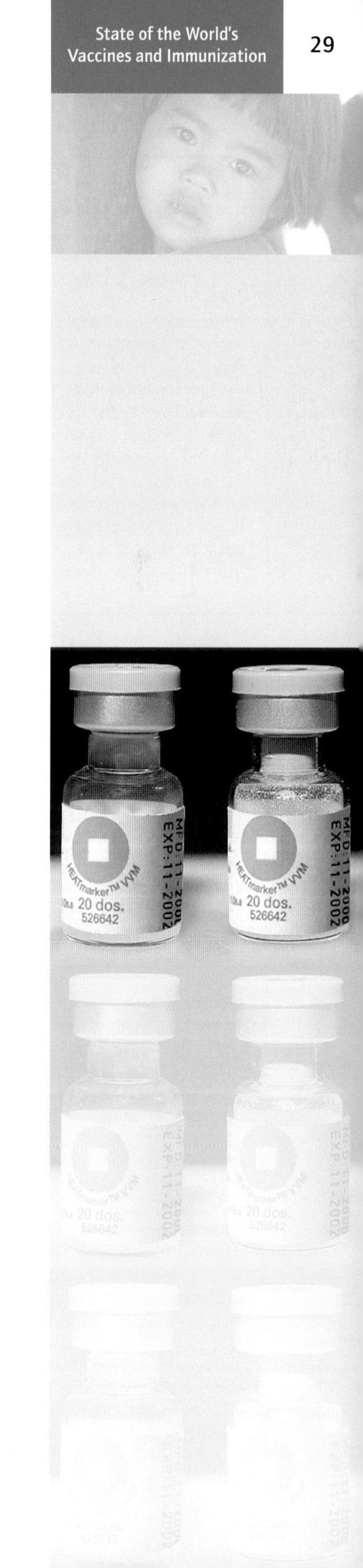

Field studies on the Uniject™ device have been conducted with community health workers in rural areas in Bolivia and in Indonesia. These showed that it could be used safely by community health workers who had previously never given injections, and could be stored in their home for extended periods without refrigeration. It is anticipated that the device will also be used in urban areas to immunize difficult-to-reach populations.

In addition, the eventual development of single-dose vaccines, combining several booster injections in one dose that would be released over time would greatly simplify immunization and solve the problem of children who fail to complete the full immunization schedule. A new single-dose TT vaccine, to replace the current three-dose regimen, is the first of these vaccines to enter clinical trials.

New initiatives on immunization safety

New global initiatives have been launched to promote and monitor immunization safety and support the development of safer vaccine technologies in response to the serious shortcomings in immunization safety identified in many developing countries.

Vaccine safety: a paradox

One of the great paradoxes of modern vaccines is that as vaccines increasingly become more effective, safe and of good quality, public concerns about their safety have tended to increase, especially in the developed world.

Alarmist reports in the medical press, often based on poor science or inadequately weighed for evidence, concern at being required to participate in national immunization programmes without freedom of choice, and the often poor handling of information by health authorities have been sufficient in many countries in Europe and North America to have an adverse effect on immunization programmes. In the UK, for example, suggestions by a small number of investigators of an association between measles-mumps-rubella (MMR) vaccine and autism (based on poor science and without foundation) has led to public concern about vaccines and immunization practices in general (see Box on Measles outbreak in the UK page 51).

Today, parents needing to get their children immunized are faced with a plethora of information from official sources as well as from the printed media, the internet, radio and television. However, disseminating this information may be confusing as the media often present information for and against a vaccine safety issue as if the pros and the cons are equal. In reality, the risk from the vaccine may be one case in a million doses given while the risk from not getting vaccinated may be one in twenty.

In recent years, WHO has taken steps to meet this modern challenge to vaccine practices. In 1997, through its International Collaborating Centre for Adverse Drug Events, WHO helped formulate the Erice Declaration which committed health authorities and practitioners to full and frank public disclosure of matters relating to drug and vaccine safety.

In 1999, WHO established an independent panel of experts in vaccine safety to advise on all vaccine safety issues. The Global Advisory Committee on Vaccine Safety also assesses the implications of these vaccine safety issues for vaccine practices worldwide and for WHO policies. To date, the committee has considered more than 20 major safety issues with potential implications for global immunization policy.

In addition, WHO has trained key health personnel responsible for national immunization policies and vaccine regulation on issues including vaccine safety, monitoring and dealing with adverse events following immunization (AEFI), as well as how to deal openly and fully with the media on vaccine safety issues. WHO has worked with more than 100 countries to improve the competence of drug regulatory personnel in evaluating and monitoring vaccine safety, quality and efficacy issues.

In this way it is hoped that trust will be restored in the effectiveness, good quality and high safety record of modern vaccines, thereby ensuring that vaccines can fulfil their public health potential.

In 1999, WHO forged a new global partnership aimed at improving immunization safety worldwide. The Immunization Safety Priority Project brings together national governments, UNICEF, UNAIDS, the World Bank Group, PATH, the Children's Vaccine Program, industry, development agencies and professional organizations. By 2003, it aims to ensure the safety of all immunizations. The project promotes the concept of the safely immunized child through efforts to ensure the safety of vaccines and injections, as well as the safe management of waste disposal. It is also supporting the development of safer vaccine delivery systems for use in developing countries.

In view of the very small proportion of injections related to immunization (less than 10%), efforts to ensure the safety of immunization injections are handled in the broader context of injection safety. The Immunization Safety Priority Project participates in the Safe Injection Global Network (SIGN) alliance, established in 1999 to ensure the safe and appropriate use of all injections worldwide. SIGN aims to prevent transmission of blood-borne diseases by reducing the number of unnecessary injections, and ensuring injection safety (including immunization injections) as well as safe waste disposal.

Assuring vaccine quality and safety

The quality of vaccines – from the production process, transport and storage of the vaccine, right up to administration – is a critical safety issue. By nature, vaccines are biologically variable. They must be produced under conditions which ensure that each batch of the product consistently shows the characteristics that are essential to its safety and efficacy. The vaccine manufacturer is responsible for product quality and most countries require an independent assessment of vaccine quality through an agency known as the National Regulatory Authority (NRA), (see Fig.9).

Since the mid-1990s, WHO has been involved in efforts to strengthen the capacity of NRAs to assess the quality and safety of vaccines used within a country – whether produced domestically or imported from elsewhere. The aim is to ensure that all countries have access to vaccines of assured quality and that the quality is maintained up to the time the vaccine is administered.

WHO has identified six key functions which NRAs must exercise in order to guarantee the quality and safety of a vaccine. These include:

- A published set of clear requirements for licensing (of products and manufacturers)
- Surveillance of vaccine field performance (safety and efficacy)
- A system of lot release
- The use of a laboratory when needed
- Regular inspections of manufacturers for compliance with Good Manufacturing Practices (GMP)
- Evaluation of clinical performance through authorized clinical trials.

In addition, there must be no unresolved confirmed reports of quality-related problems. Countries that produce their own vaccines are required to exercise all six functions, while those that import vaccines have a reduced role since some of the functions (e.g. inspection for compliance with GMP) will already have been carried out by the NRA in the country of manufacture. Where the NRA is unable to fulfil even this reduced role, countries are advised to source their vaccines through the UNICEF procurement system, which uses the WHO prequalification system.

Figure 9: **Status of National Regulatory Authorities (NRAs) June 2002**

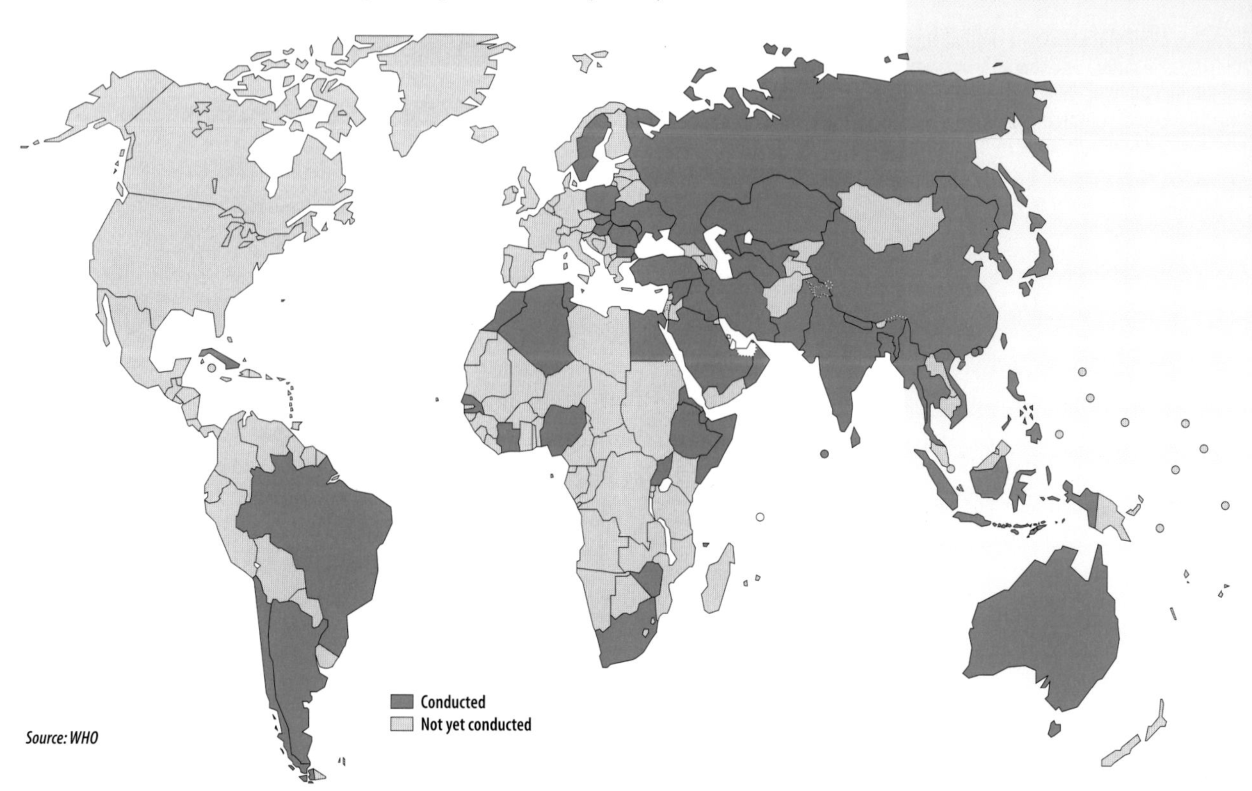

Source: WHO

In 1996, a Global Training Network was established to provide training in the regulation of vaccines for staff from NRAs, national immunization programmes and vaccine manufacturers. And since 1997, regular assessments have been carried out by teams of experts to determine whether the NRA is performing a set of essential regulation functions for vaccine. If the NRA is failing in one or more areas, technical support and training needs are identified and staff are offered a placement on a network training course. Within 12 months, a follow-up assessment is carried out to re-evaluate the performance of the NRA, and re-assessments are carried out every two years to ensure that standards are being maintained.

The original network of five training centres has expanded to 13 and over 460 staff from 76 countries have received training. A new course on regulatory issues in vaccine procurement is now also provided for regulatory staff.

In addition to ensuring vaccine quality at the outset, there is an urgent need to strengthen training and supervision of vaccine transport, storage and administration, in order to ensure that vaccine is safe and potent right up to the moment it is administered to a child. WHO has developed guidelines and training courses for health workers to ensure that procedures are correctly followed and to minimize the risk of programme errors.

Thiomersal in children's vaccines

In the late 1990s, concerns were raised in the USA about the safety of thiomersal - a preservative used in some vaccines - and containing ethyl-mercury. This was based on the realization that the cumulative amount of mercury in the infant immunization schedule potentially exceeded the recommended threshold for exposure to methyl-mercury set by one of the US government agencies. This latter compound was reported to cause neurological abnormalities in newborns following foetal exposure after ingestion by the pregnant mother of large doses over a long period of time.

As a result of this theoretical concern, a recommendation to expedite removal of thiomersal from vaccines was made in 1999 by the two US immunization related advisory bodies. This decision has put pressure on other countries to follow the lead of the US. The removal of thiomersal, however, may lead to changes in vaccine potency, stability and reactogenicity, and needs to be done with great caution.

Since the decision was taken in the US, reassuring additional information has become available. In particular, it was shown that the pharmacokinetic profile of ethyl-mercury is very different from that of methyl-mercury and rapidly excreted through the gut. In addition, several epidemiologic studies recently completed have been reassuring with respect to the safety of thiomersal contained in vaccines.

Two independent expert groups, the Global Advisory Committee on Vaccine Safety and the US Institute of Medicine, have reviewed the issue and have found no scientific evidence of toxicity from thiomersal containing vaccines. As a result, the WHO Strategic Advisory Group of Experts (SAGE), at its June 2002 meeting, strongly affirmed that vaccines containing thiomersal should continue to be used for maintaining safe immunization.

Thiomersal has been used for over 60 years as an antimicrobial (preservative) agent in vaccines and other pharmaceutical products to prevent unwanted growth of microorganisms. No other preservative with a similar safety profile is as effective as thiomersal. In vaccines, there is a specific need for preservatives for multi-dose presentations of vaccines such as DTP (diphtheria-tetanus-pertussis), tetanus toxoid, hepatitis B and *Haemophilus influenzae* type b. The repeated puncture of the rubber stopper and further withdrawing of vaccine poses a risk of contamination and related transmission to the children. Thiomersal cannot be removed without threatening and potentiallly compromising the quality of childhood vaccines used in global programmes. Live vaccines, bacterial or viral vaccines such as that for measles, do not contain preservatives as they would interfere with the active ingredients. Over the years, thiomersal has prevented illness and death by reducing the risk of contamination of opened multi-dose vials. In certain vaccines, thiomersal is also used during the manufacturing process.

Safer injections

As evidence has emerged of the vast scale of unsafe injection practices in the developing world and the high death toll involved, efforts to improve injection safety have been intensified. In 1999, a joint statement was issued by WHO, UNICEF, UNFPA and the IFRC, urging all donors who finance vaccines to adopt the so-called "bundling policy" – supplying all vaccines together with AD syringes (designed to prevent re-use) and puncture-proof safety boxes for safe waste disposal. They also recommended that standard disposable syringes and needles should no longer be used for immunization and that the use of sterilizable syringes should be phased out by 2003.

This policy has been adopted by GAVI, which is committed to supplying all vaccines complete with AD syringes and safety boxes. In addition, countries applying for support through GAVI are required to develop an injection safety plan as part of their application to the Vaccine Fund. To help countries assess the safety of their injection and disposal practices, an assessment tool has been developed jointly by WHO, SIGN and Basic Support for Institutionalizing Child Survival (BASICS), a USAID-funded programme. A team monitors injection practices in 80 centres in 10 districts over two weeks, using direct observation, stock control and interview techniques.

In 2001, about 600 million AD syringes were distributed for use in developing countries around the world. By 2003, that number is expected to rise to well over 1.5 billion, dramatically increasing the hazardous waste that has to be incinerated or buried. WHO has produced guidelines on the management of health care waste including injection equipment. Countries are advised to establish a national policy for safe health-care waste management; to establish legal and financial responsibility (including regulations and guidelines); to provide training; and to select a waste disposal system that is safe, environmentally friendly and sustainable.

The price of AD syringes has fallen as their use has increased, and could fall even further following the transfer of technology for local production in countries including China, India, Malaysia, Russia and Viet Nam. When used correctly, the AD syringe offers the lowest risk of blood-borne transmission of diseases. But continued efforts are also needed to train and motivate health workers, encourage behaviour change and educate people to insist on the use of a sterile syringe for every injection.

In the longer-term, technological advances such as needle-free devices and new kinds of vaccines have the potential to further greatly improve injection safety. These include: needle-free jet guns designed to give a rapid series of injections, one after the other; sugar glass vaccines, in which dry powder vaccine is released when the sugar glass ("needle") comes into contact with water or body fluids; nasal vaccines; new oral vaccines; skin patch vaccines, in which vaccine is absorbed through the skin; and edible vaccines in which vaccines are produced and delivered in genetically-engineered fruit and vegetables.

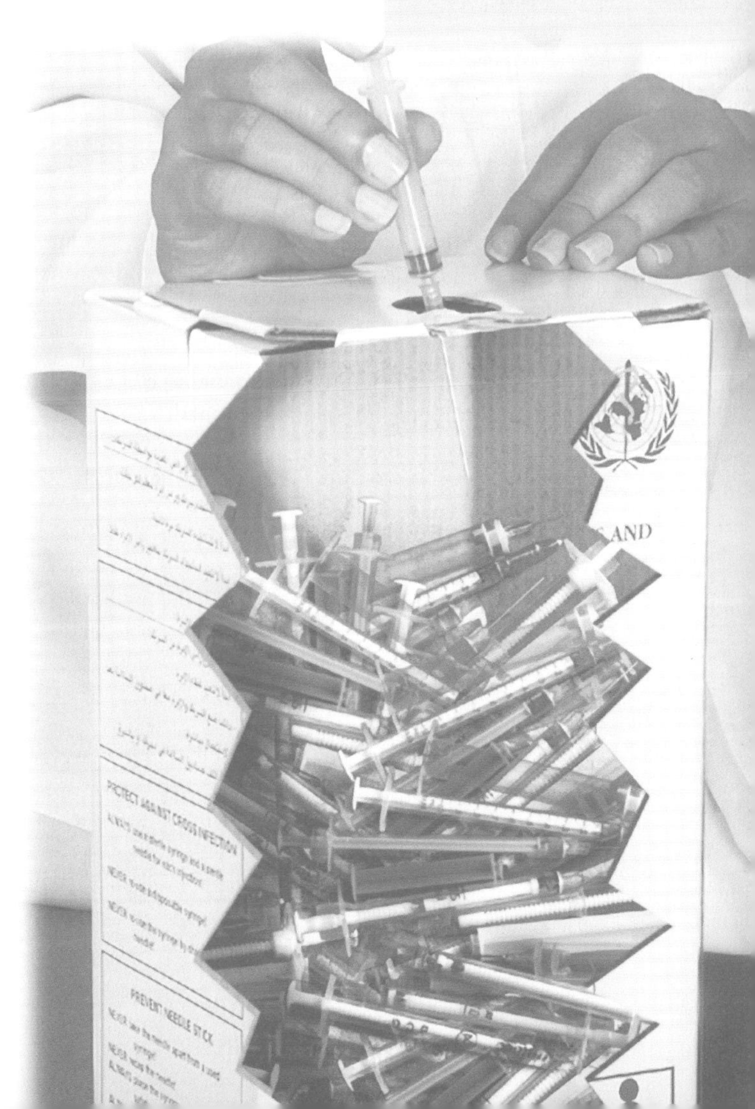

4. Financing vaccines and immunization

This section underlines the critical need to increase the financing of immunization in developing countries and looks at a range of potential new financing mechanisms. While national governments will continue to have the main responsibility for financing their national immunization programmes, low-income countries are not expected to become self-sufficient in the short- to medium-term. In the meantime, international donors are being urged to increase their funding for immunization to help fill the gaps.

Mobilizing increased financing of immunization

National governments in both developing and developed countries have the primary responsibility to assure the sustainable financing of their national immunization programme. However, as routine immunization coverage has fallen in many of the poorest countries and newer vaccines remain out of reach for the children who need them most, there is a growing consensus that increased financing of immunization is also a shared global responsibility. This new understanding is captured in the GAVI definition of sustainable financing for immunization. This definition makes it clear that, while self-sufficiency remains the ultimate goal for all countries, in the short term the measure of financial sustainability is a country's ability to mobilize both domestic and external funding on a reliable basis and to use the funds efficiently to achieve immunization targets (see Fig.10).

Today there is a renewed interest in channeling funds to immunization programmes. The Vaccine Fund and GAVI partners, including the World Bank (through loans and credits) and large foundations, are mobilizing national and international funds for immunization. GAVI partners are working with governments to increase the level of funding available, while taking steps to avoid the aid dependency that characterized the 1980s. Governments are being encouraged to take on a coordinating role. They are being urged to assume overall responsibility for securing sustainable funding for their vaccine needs from both domestic and external resources, and for using those resources as efficiently as possible. In return for external support, they are also required to meet standards for quality and safety, to reach increasing numbers of hard-to-reach children and to take steps to ensure sustainable financing. This new approach depends on strong government commitment to

Figure 10: **Variability in sources of financing of immunization programmes for selected countries***

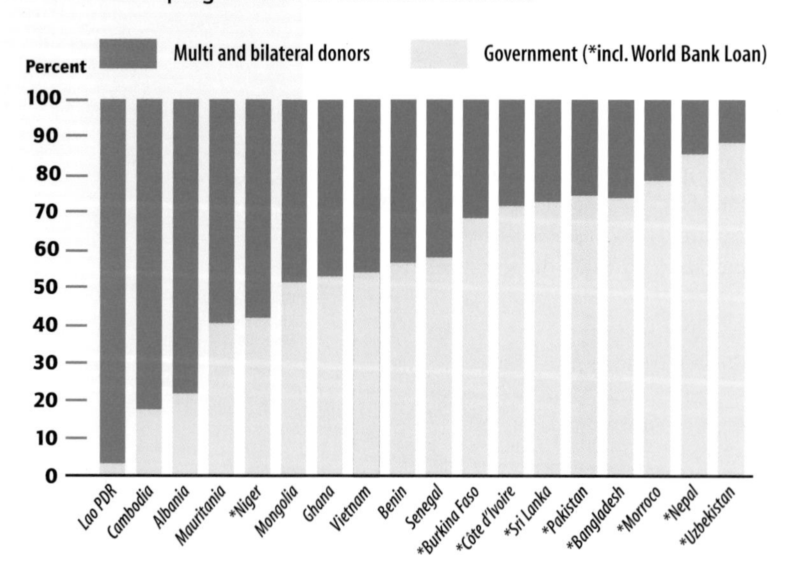

Source: GAVI Financing Task Force
**based on recent country financing assessments done between 1998 and 2001*

immunization, backed up by good evidence (e.g. estimates of the cost-effectiveness of vaccines compared to other health interventions) in order to argue the case powerfully with decision-makers.

Every year, about US$ 1.56 billion of external assistance is provided for immunization in developing countries, of which about US$ 1.1 billion is spent in low-income countries. In 1999, GAVI looked at overall spending on immunization in the poorest countries and set out to estimate how much more it would cost to reach the millions of children with no access to traditional EPI vaccines or under-used vaccines such as hepatitis B and Hib.

It was estimated that, with an additional investment of about US$ 250 million a year in low-income countries, at least 10 million more children could be reached with the traditional EPI vaccines by 2005. To reach the same number of children with additional vaccines against hepatitis B and Hib will cost about US$ 350 million more each year.

National funding commitments

Governments in developing countries are being urged by WHO, UNICEF, the World Bank Group and others to increase their spending on immunization, as part of a larger effort to reorient public spending to the interventions, services and programmes that are cost-effective, and for which the public sector has primary responsibility. Depending on the context, a variety of approaches can be taken by a country to move towards a higher level of spending on immunization – and a better return on every dollar, peso, shilling or baht spent. These include:

- **Use of cost-effectiveness and public finance principles to allocate funding:** Moving away from a situation in which resource allocation is based on political imperatives and towards an evidence-based approach can only benefit the immunization programme and the long-term aims of the health system as a whole. This implies setting priorities based on a combination of cost-effectiveness analyses that are appropriate to the epidemiological and economic context of the country and an understanding of the core responsibilities of the government as a financier of services that have social benefits.

- **Establishment of legal mandates for baseline funding of national immunization programmes:** This would attempt to reduce the erratic nature of public funding and guarantee at least the bare minimum of support, regardless of the political climate or competing needs. Achieving this requires strong political support and clear arguments to distinguish the immunization programme from other health services.

- **Using immunization coverage and other measures of programme performance as indicators of public health system performance:** When governments use quantitative targets for immunization programme performance within their health sector strategic plans, national development plans, poverty reduction strategies or other major statements of high-level goals, they are indicating that immunization is a priority, and that they are committed to making every effort to secure funding. Knowing that they will be reporting on progress toward those targets in the future can be a powerful motivating force to both politicians and bureaucrats. Setting targets, and reporting on progress toward them, at the district level can have the same effect in decentralized systems, where at least some of the funding decisions are made by provincial and/or district authorities.

- **Taking steps to make sure that funding is used efficiently:** In highly resource-constrained environments, the need for attention to efficiency is obvious – and presents a tremendous challenge for programme managers. Planning so that all the appropriate inputs – vaccines, syringes, personnel, vehicles, fuel and refrigerators – are in the right place at the right time minimizes wasted time and other valuable resources. Streamlining bureaucratic processes so that information about funding needs and use of funds flow smoothly, and funds are disbursed in a timely manner, often permits programmes to achieve much higher levels of performance with no net increase in the financial resources required. And, importantly, a smoothly running, efficient programme is likely to attract and retain support from both domestic and international sources.

- **Working with external financiers (including donor and lending agencies) to determine strategic, predictable levels of support:** The international community increasingly recognizes that, for the lowest-income countries, large improvements in immunization coverage and the introduction of new and underused vaccines will only be feasible with external support. The challenge is to ensure that the external support is directed toward key inputs in a way that does not displace domestic investment, yet that in fact stimulates greater levels of national funding in the long-term.

The Bill & Melinda Gates Foundation

The Bill & Melinda Gates Foundation is dedicated to improving people's lives by sharing advances in health and learning with the global community. The foundation was created in January of 2000, through the merger of the Gates Learning Foundation, which focused on expanding access to technology through public libraries, and the William H. Gates Foundation, which focused on improving global health. Led by Bill Gates' father, William H. Gates, Sr., and Patty Stonesifer, the Seattle-based foundation has an endowment of approximately $24 billion. The foundation's Global Health Program is focused on reducing global health inequities by accelerating the development, deployment and sustainability of health interventions that will save lives and dramatically reduce the disease burden in developing countries.

"The opportunity to eliminate the vaccine gap has never been greater. Through funding, leadership and collaboration, we can ensure that vaccines are available to every child, everywhere. But to reach this goal, substantial increases in public investment and new market incentives are needed to lower prices of existing vaccines and spur the development of new vaccines such as HIV/AIDS, tuberculosis and malaria. Today, only 10% of the world's health resources are devoted to addressing the diseases that make up 90% of the world's health problems. Clearly, world governments must step up their investment in a dramatic way."

Patty Stonesifer
Co-chair and President
Bill & Melinda Gates Foundation

New financing mechanisms

In addition to urging countries to maximize traditional sources of funding, GAVI partners are also involved in efforts to identify innovative new financial strategies that can be used to fund immunization and the development of priority new vaccines for developing countries.

One promising source of additional funding is the use of debt relief funds. Debt relief for the countries most burdened by debt – through the Heavily Indebted Poor Countries (HIPC) Initiative – could boost domestic financing of vaccines if immunization is well positioned within countries' poverty reduction strategies. About 30 countries are currently eligible for support through the HIPC Initiative, a World Bank programme designed to obtain debt relief (subject to satisfactory policy performance) and ensure that structural adjustment and reform efforts are not compromised by the continuing burden of high debt repayments. The HIPC Initiative can reduce debt servicing substantially, allowing the savings to be allocated to social expenditure, such as primary health care, basic education, or improving water supplies and sanitation. In Uganda, for example, the first country to receive HIPC funding, the debt relief was used to boost primary school enrolment.

Another possibility being explored by a few small countries is the establishment of a national trust fund. This is a flexible funding mechanism set up with a financial endowment and clear policy aims. On a national level, a trust fund earmarked for immunization could provide a reliable flow of funds over a long period, protected from the politics of annual budgeting.

Soft loans (or concessionary credits) – a form of borrowing subsidized by development banks for the lowest-income countries – are another potential source of funding for immunization. The main lender for immunization is the World Bank, but regional development banks, such as the Asian Development Bank, also finance immunization. The World Bank makes soft loans – known as International Development Association (IDA) loans – available to poorer countries that meet certain economic management and policy conditions. Loan conditions need to balance accountability with flexibility. Countries pay no interest, repayment periods can be as long as 40 years and borrowers pay only an administrative fee of slightly less than 1% of the loan's value. Given the long payback time, the loan is given at a significant discount, currently estimated at 65% grant, 35% pay back. In addition, the World Bank has recently approved an IDA grant facility making new funds available to the poorest countries.

With adequate investment there is renewed hope that the promise of immunization can be realized for children throughout the world. GAVI is today providing the catalyst needed to reverse the decline in immunization, accelerate the introduction of new vaccines in developing countries and secure immunization at the heart of development efforts. In addition, other organizations and development partners around the world are working to put an end to the unacceptable status quo in immunization and establish a new, more equitable system for the world's children. END Part 2

Investment Partnership for Polio (IDA "buy-downs")

This novel funding mechanism is a way of providing governments with additional financial resources in the form of soft loans (IDA), without the usual repayment obligations. Initially focused on polio eradication projects, it is being piloted with the support of the Gates Foundation, Rotary International and the United Nations Foundation. The partnership is an example of innovative approaches from the World Bank which are aimed at improving the delivery of global public goods, in particular those related to the control of communicable diseases.

Under this new funding mechanism, IDA credits (low interest loans) will be approved for countries to purchase OPV. At the same time, third party funding will also be mobilized to "buy down", or cover, the service charge and repayments. In this way, countries can access what is in essence grant funding to eradicate polio. The benefits of this investment will extend beyond national borders, eliminating the risk that people in other polio-free countries will become infected.

Mobilization of third party funding for this Investment Partnership for Polio is well under way. The Gates Foundation, Rotary International and the United Nations Foundation have committed US$ 50 million, an amount that will enable the World Bank to provide US$ 130–150 million in IDA funding on a grant basis for polio eradication.

Part 3: Vaccines update

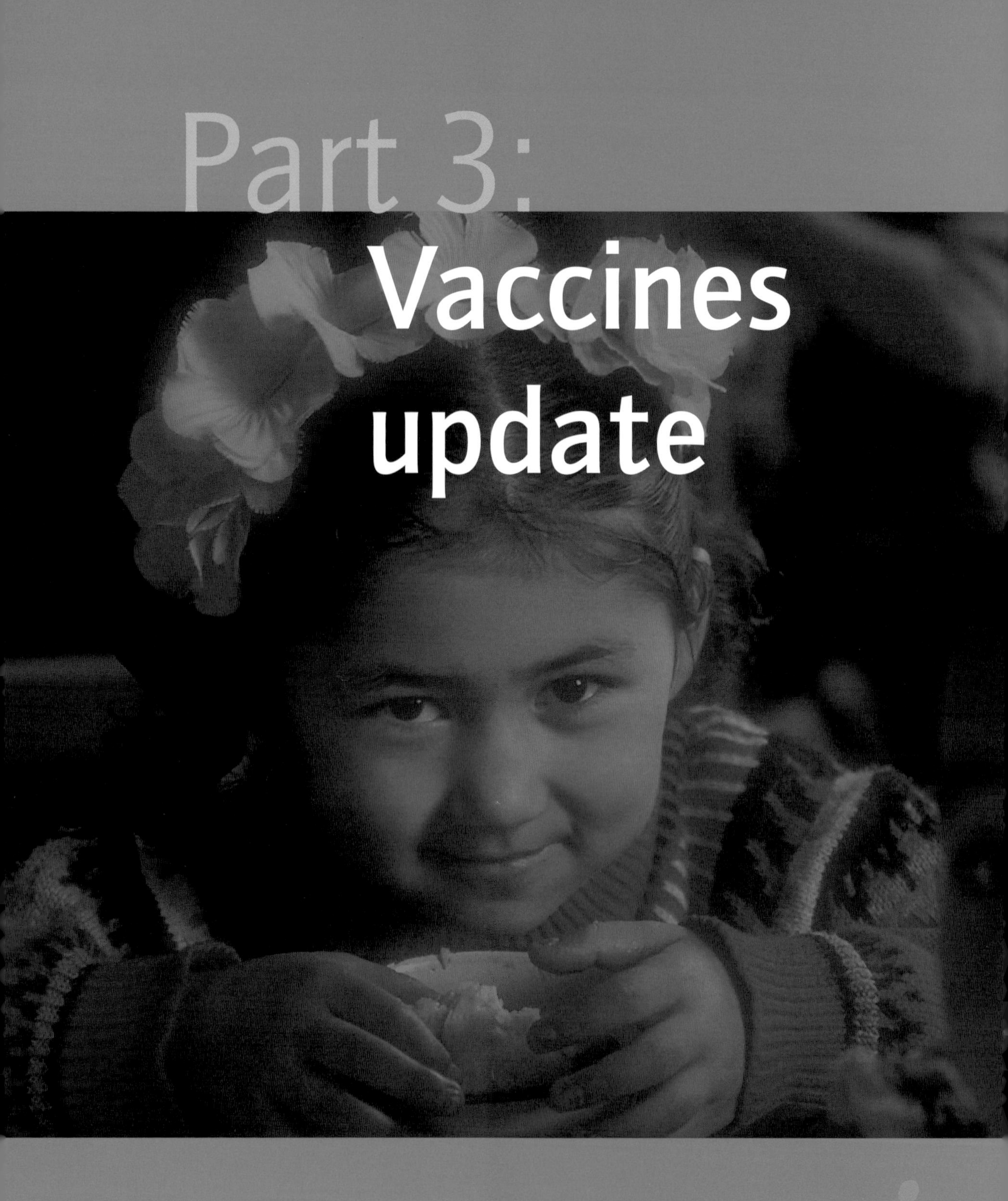

Part 3

looks at the impact of some vaccines already in use today and reviews progress in the research and development (R&D) of priority new vaccines for developing countries.

s save lives

1. Under-used vaccines

- ***Haemophilus influenzae*** **type b**
- **Hepatitis B**
- **Yellow fever**
- **Rubella**

By the end of 2001, 142 states and territories were using hepatitis B vaccine in their routine infant immunization programmes (almost 75% of countries)

Four existing vaccines– against *Haemophilus influenzae* type b (Hib), hepatitis B, yellow fever and rubella – are still not available today in many of the countries where they are needed most.

Since 1997, WHO has recommended that the Hib conjugate vaccine, which was developed over a decade ago, should be included in routine infant immunization schedules, wherever resources are available and control of the disease is a priority (based on disease burden data). Both prerequisites – adequate resources and awareness of disease burden for decision-making – have been difficult to achieve in low-income countries and the uptake of the vaccine in the developing world has generally been slow. However, the situation is now changing. Hib vaccine has recently been introduced in most Latin American countries and in an increasing number of countries in the Middle East and Africa. By 2001, 90 countries had introduced the vaccine. GAVI has set a target for the use of Hib vaccine: 50% of the least-developed countries with a high disease burden and adequate delivery systems should have introduced Hib vaccine in routine immunization schedules by 2005.

In 1992, the World Health Assembly recommended that all countries with a high disease burden should introduce hepatitis B vaccine in their routine infant immunization programmes by 1995 and all countries by 1997. A year later, an additional target was added – an 80% reduction in the incidence of new hepatitis B carriers among children by 2001. But uptake of the vaccine has been slow and the targets have not been met. By the end of 2001, 142 states and territories were using hepatitis B vaccine in their routine infant immunization programmes (almost 75% of countries). GAVI has set a new target for hepatitis B: 80% of developing countries should have introduced the vaccine (a target expected to be met) by 2002, and all countries by 2007.

The use of yellow fever vaccine – an inexpensive vaccine available since 1937 – has largely been a public health failure. Widely deployed in disease-endemic countries from the 1950s to the 1970s, together with vector control measures, it was abandoned by cash-strapped governments (along with vector control) once the disease appeared to be under control. As a result, there has been a resurgence of yellow fever. Over the past two decades, there were 12 times as many cases as during the previous two decades. In 2001 alone there were seven outbreaks of the disease in Africa.

Since 1988, WHO has recommended that yellow fever vaccine should be included in routine immunization schedules in all high-risk countries – immunizing children from six months onwards. A single dose of the vaccine provides immunity for at least 10 years and in disease-endemic areas probably for

life. Worldwide, 44 countries today are at risk of yellow fever (33 in Africa and 11 in the Americas). Of these, 26 have so far included the vaccine in routine immunization schedules. Since the launch of GAVI, yellow fever vaccine is being made available on request in all countries at risk – regardless of their current level of DTP immunization coverage – and is financed through the Vaccine Fund.

Universal rubella immunization has not been recommended by WHO to date because of the need for countries to ensure high sustained coverage. Coverage of over 80% among children is needed to prevent a shift in the incidence of the disease to older age groups – increasing the risk of congenital rubella syndrome (CRS) due to infection during pregnancy. However, the disease has been virtually eliminated in some developed countries following the success of sustained childhood immunization programmes, usually involving the use of MMR vaccine.

Haemophilus influenzae type b

In developing countries, *Haemophilus influenzae* type b (Hib) disease kills about 450 000 children every year. Most children die from pneumonia and a minority from meningitis. The disease has virtually disappeared in the developed countries since the vaccine was introduced over a decade ago, but it continues to exert a heavy toll elsewhere.

Hib is a leading cause of pneumonia in developing countries, accounting for up to 20% of severe pneumonia in some developing countries. The bacterium also accounts for one-third to one-half of cases of bacterial meningitis in children under two years. In developing countries, about 40% of Hib meningitis cases are fatal, and 15–35% of children who survive are left with permanent disabilities such as brain damage and hearing loss. The bacterium is showing increasing resistance to antibiotics.

In the Americas, Hib conjugate vaccine has been gradually introduced over the past decade – initially in Canada and the United States, next in Uruguay and Chile, and then in other countries throughout Latin America. The vaccine has been made available through the PAHO's revolving fund. By 1999, over 80% of children were immunized and the incidence of the disease had fallen dramatically. During 2002, 93% of countries throughout Latin America and the Caribbean are expected to be using the vaccine in routine immunization programmes. As the market expanded during the 1990s, the price of the vaccine for countries in the region fell from US$ 6–8 per dose in 1997 to US$ 2.18–2.60 in 1999. By 2002, the lowest available price for countries eligible to buy vaccines through the UNICEF procurement system was US$ 2.65 per dose of monovalent lyophilized (freeze-dried) Hib in a one-dose vial or US$ 3.25 for a two-dose vial of combined DTP-HepB-Hib vaccine. Three doses of the vaccine are needed during the first year of life starting from the age of six weeks.

In other parts of the developing world, uptake of Hib vaccine has been slower. Despite the recent introduction of the vaccine in a number of countries in Africa

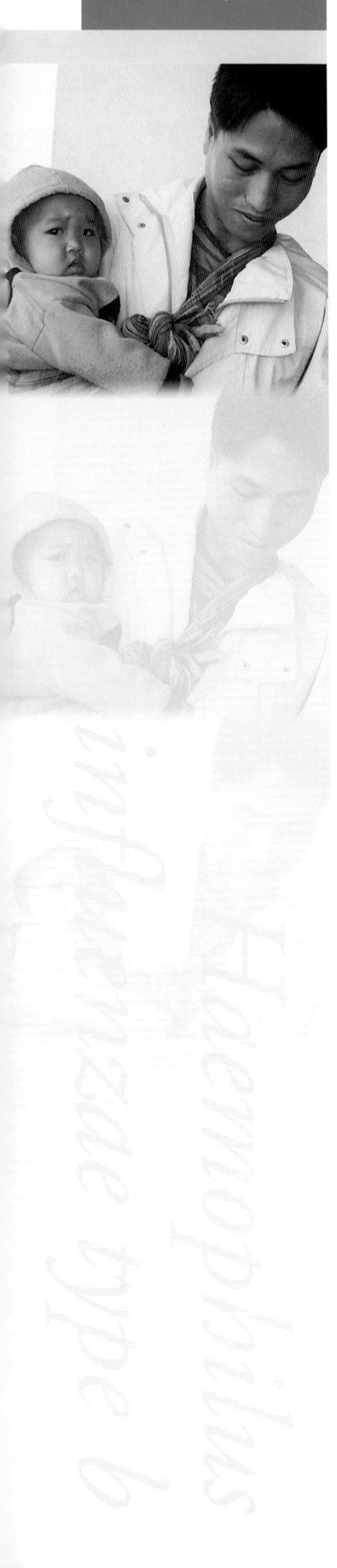

and the Middle East, by 2001, only one in five children worldwide were immunized against Hib disease during the first year of life. Of the 90 countries using the vaccine in routine immunization programmes, most were high- or middle-income countries. Only 5% of countries with a per capita GNP of less than US$ 1000 had introduced the vaccine, compared with 75% of countries with a per capita GNP greater than US$ 12 000. Since then, the Vaccine Fund has approved funding for Hib vaccine for 11 of the least-developed countries which requested support for this vaccine (as of March 2002).

One reason for the low uptake of Hib vaccine in developing countries outside Latin America, apart from the relatively high price, is the lack of data on disease burden and the difficulty in assessing it. Pneumonia and meningitis are frequently caused by other microbes and accurate diagnosis can be difficult (e.g. for meningitis, a lumbar puncture is needed followed by laboratory analysis). Many low-income countries lack the facilities needed to carry out these kind of analyses. The precise cause of pneumonia is more difficult to determine, even with the best laboratory support. As a result, the burden of Hib disease is not well documented and doctors, even if they do treat this disease, fail to identify the cause.

To help countries assess the disease burden and the potential cost-effectiveness of introducing the vaccine more accurately, WHO, the Centers for Disease Control and Prevention (CDC) and other partners, have developed a rapid assessment tool which can produce nationwide estimates of the Hib disease burden within 10 days. These estimates are based on assessments carried out in several districts. This involves the use of clinical and laboratory records for all meningitis cases in order to estimate the proportion of cases attributable to Hib. This is then used to estimate the number of severe Hib pneumonia cases (about five times the meningitis cases). The number of Hib deaths is extrapolated from the total number of deaths from acute respiratory infections among children under five.

Meanwhile other studies are being undertaken in a number of countries to establish the Hib disease burden and assess the impact and cost-effectiveness of introducing the vaccine. In Tunisia, efforts are also under way to establish a surveillance system to monitor the impact of the introduction of Hib vaccine. In the Gambia, the first African country to introduce Hib vaccine, WHO is supporting a study on the impact of the vaccine on the immunization programme and on the disease burden, while in Brazil and Colombia, WHO is supporting an evaluation of the impact of Hib vaccine on the incidence of pneumonia.

In an effort to develop local surveillance capacity, WHO has established a network for surveillance of laboratory-confirmed bacterial meningitis among children, funded by the Children's Vaccine Program and USAID. Launched in 2001, initially in sub-Saharan Africa, this initiative is providing each country with US$ 14 000 for training and equipment. Work is currently under way to expand the network to countries in North Africa and the Middle East.

Hepatitis B

Up to 100 times more infectious than HIV, hepatitis B is second only to tobacco as a recognized cause of a major cancer in humans. In 2000, there were an estimated 5.2 million cases of acute hepatitis B infection and over 520 000 deaths from hepatitis B-related diseases (almost 470 000 from cirrhosis and liver cancer and 52 000 from acute hepatitis B).

About one-third of the world's population (around 2 billion people) are believed to have been infected with the virus at some time during their lifetime. Of these, over 350 million people are chronically infected carriers of the disease – most of them infected at birth or during early childhood. Primary liver cancer is the main cause of cancer deaths among men in sub-Saharan Africa and much of Asia, and an important cause of cancer deaths among women worldwide. Hepatitis B infection accounts for 60–80% of primary liver cancer worldwide.

Up to 100 times more infectious than HIV, hepatitis B is second only to tobacco as a recognized cause of a major cancer in humans

Mother-to-child and child-to-child transmission accounts for the majority of infections and carriers. Although young children rarely develop the acute form of the disease, at least one in four of those infected before the age of seven will become long-term carriers – with no sign of illness until much later in life. The disease is also transmitted through the use of unsterile needles or other medical equipment, unsafe blood transfusions, unprotected sex and cultural practices which involve skin piercing.

The "invisibility" of the chronic form of the disease is one of the reasons why the disease has been neglected for so long in developing countries. The initial high price of the vaccine is another. When the vaccine first became available over 20 years ago it cost US$ 150 for three doses, 150 times more than the total cost of all six traditional EPI vaccines then in use. Its arrival on the market signalled an end to the "cheap vaccine era" and helped focus global attention on the increasing inequity in access to vaccines and immunization. The failure to attract national government funding and increased donor support for hepatitis B vaccine in the worst affected countries, even when the price fell substantially, was a warning of what might happen to other new vaccines urgently needed today in developing countries. As a result, from the mid-1990s onwards, the fate of hepatitis B vaccine became a catalyst for change. Today, it is one of the three priority vaccines which is being made available to the poorest countries for five years through the Vaccine Fund. In 2002, the lowest available price for countries eligible to buy vaccines through the UNICEF procurement system was US$ 0.25– 0.43 (10-dose vial).

By the end of 2001, 142 countries were using hepatitis B vaccine in routine infant immunization schedules (see Fig.11). Over 40 of the least-developed countries are currently being funded through the Vaccine Fund for the introduction of hepatitis B vaccine in routine schedules (as of March 2002).

Figure 11: **Number of countries introduced HepB vaccine and global HepB3 coverage*, 1989-2001**

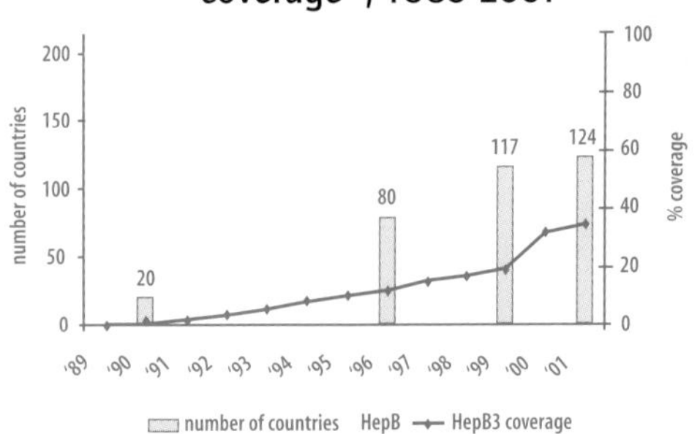

*3 consecutive doses of HepB vaccine by age 6 months

Source:WHO/UNICEF joint reporting form, 2001 & WHO country information, 2001

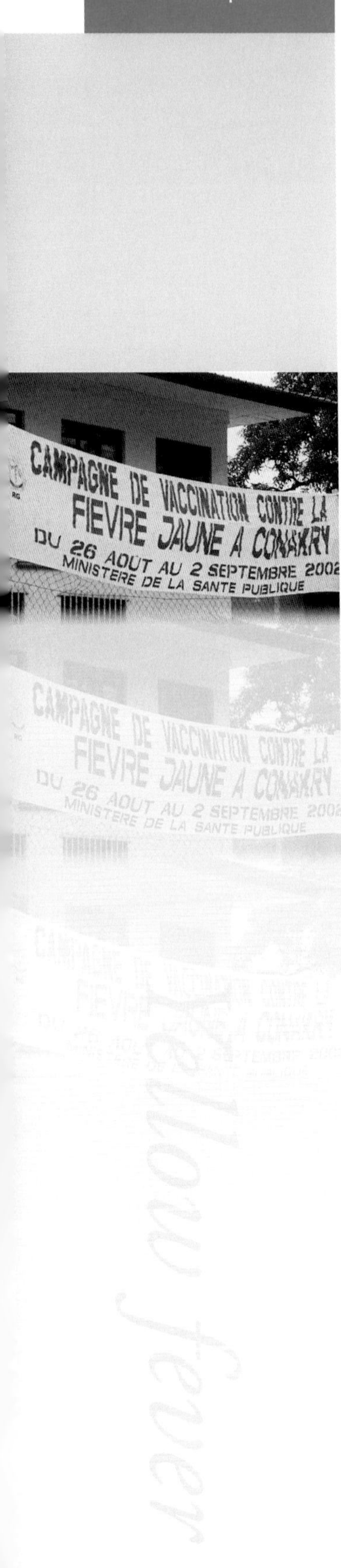

Yellow fever

Yellow fever is a re-emerging viral haemorrhagic fever which occurs, often in explosive epidemics, in parts of Africa and the Americas with heavy loss of life. A disease that once plagued Europe and North America, yellow fever has the potential to spread beyond its present range – into Asia, for example – wherever the mosquito vector exists. Every year there are an estimated 200 000 cases of yellow fever and about 30 000 deaths, of which only a tiny fraction are reported. No specific antiviral drugs exist to treat the disease.

In tropical forested areas, where monkeys act as a reservoir for the virus, yellow fever circulates at a low level all the time, often affecting migrant workers such as loggers. But when the virus is introduced into a densely populated urban area, it can spark off a major epidemic.

This would not happen if most people were vaccinated, but immunization coverage and mosquito control activities fell sharply during the 1970s, after widespread use of the vaccine appeared to have brought the disease under control. Many of the countries where yellow fever is endemic are among the poorest in the world, and when the disease appeared to be under control both governments and donors turned their attention to the control of other diseases which posed a more immediate and visible threat.

Of the 37 countries at high risk for yellow fever, 26 (70%) have included the vaccine in their routine immunization programmes. However, while coverage in the Americas is good, it is generally poor in Africa, due in part to lack of awareness of the disease burden and lack of resources for preventive immunization campaigns. At the same time, mosquito populations and habitats have increased and the mobility of people to and from endemic areas is more frequent today. To further complicate matters, a recent resurgence of yellow fever coincided with a temporary shortage of the vaccine, which was the result of the fall-off in demand and the low profitability of the vaccine.

During 2001, efforts to respond to outbreaks of yellow fever in Africa were hampered by the vaccine shortage and the lack of an emergency stockpile. A large outbreak in Guinea in 2000 involving over 800 cases and almost 250 deaths depleted global stocks of the vaccine. This in turn lead to the establishment of an emergency stockpile. This mechanism is operated by the International Coordinating Group on Vaccine Provision, established in 1997 in response to a crisis in the supply of meningitis vaccine for use in epidemics. During 2001, UNICEF supplied 2 million doses of yellow fever vaccine for emergency use through this mechanism. It has yet to be decided how big the stockpile should be, how it will be replenished and how it will be funded in future. Although there is no longer a global shortage of yellow fever vaccine for routine immunization and preventive campaigns, the problem of supply arises during outbreaks when large amounts of vaccine are needed at very short notice.

In 2001, an outbreak of yellow fever in Abidjan, Côte d'Ivoire – the first urban outbreak in Africa for a decade – was a test of the effectiveness of the new mechanism. WHO launched an urgent appeal to the international community for almost US$ 3 million to finance a mass immunization campaign, including the purchase of vaccine from the emergency stockpile. Over 90% of the population were immunized over 10 days, averting what could have been a humanitarian disaster.

By October 2001, the outbreak had been contained to 55 suspected cases and seven deaths. This was the result of good surveillance and a rapid emergency response by WHO and other partners in the Global Outbreak Alert and Emergency Response Network. Yet if a second urban epidemic had surfaced elsewhere, the outcome would have been very different. During the outbreak in Abidjan, over 2.6 million doses of vaccine were needed to contain the epidemic in a single city. When it was over, the emergency stockpile had been exhausted. It is now estimated that a stockpile of 5 million doses may be required in future to meet emergency needs.

Immunization coverage of at least 80% nationwide is needed to prevent epidemics of yellow fever

However, emergency response is expensive. It disrupts fragile health care delivery systems and places enormous strain on both human and financial resources. It is also far less cost-effective than routine delivery of the vaccine through the EPI. A study in Nigeria in the 1990s showed that routine immunization was seven times more cost-effective. WHO recommends four strategies for the prevention and control of yellow fever:

- i) Routine immunization from nine months and mass campaigns in high-risk areas
- ii) Strengthened surveillance, including laboratory capacity to confirm suspected cases
- iii) Strengthened outbreak response through inter-country planning and improved epidemic preparedness
- iv) Efforts to assure a sustainable supply of vaccines.

In the Gambia, for example, a mass immunization campaign was launched in response to a yellow fever outbreak in 1978-79. All age groups above six months were vaccinated. In order to avoid a build-up of unvaccinated populations in future, the campaign was immediately followed by the introduction of the vaccine in the childhood immunization programme. By 2000, 85% of children were immunized against the disease and there have been no reported cases of yellow fever among Gambians since the last epidemic ended in 1979.

Immunization coverage of at least 80% nationwide is needed to prevent epidemics of yellow fever. In order to reach this level, preventive mass campaigns are needed to immunize older groups as well. Without a comprehensive campaign strategy, it would take decades to build up enough protective immunity through routine childhood immunization alone. Of the seven countries that had yellow fever outbreaks in 2001, only four had included the vaccine in their routine programme and none had carried out preventive campaigns in high-risk areas.

GAVI is making yellow fever vaccine available for routine immunization wherever requested in countries where the disease is endemic. However, of the 32 African countries eligible for support for yellow fever vaccine, only 10 have applied so far. Of these, six have been approved for funding through the Vaccine Fund (as of March 2002). Yellow fever vaccine is available through UNICEF at US$ 0.50-0.84 per dose (including the cost of syringes and safety boxes).

Rubella (German measles)

Rubella normally occurs as a mild rash disease that mainly affects children. However, if the viral disease is contracted during early pregnancy, 90% of cases result in foetal death or CRS involving multiple disabilities, including heart defects, brain damage, blindness and deafness. It is estimated that there are over 100 000 cases of CRS a year worldwide. The cost of caring for children with CRS is high, even in developing countries. Cost-benefit studies of rubella vaccination, carried out in both developing and developed countries with high immunization coverage (over 80%), have demonstrated that the benefits outweigh the costs, particularly when rubella vaccine is combined with measles vaccine.

The primary target group for rubella vaccination is women of childbearing age (15-40 years), and this strategy should ideally be combined with childhood immunization. However, large-scale rubella vaccination of children is only recommended where coverage of at least 80% can be achieved. Where coverage is lower, or not sustained, reduced circulation of rubella in the community can lead to a shift in the incidence of disease towards older age groups, increasing the risks for women of childbearing age.

Most developed countries include rubella vaccine in their national immunization programmes, usually administered in the second year of life as a combined measles-mumps-rubella (MMR) vaccine, instead of monovalent measles vaccine. Some countries also give a second dose of MMR vaccine at school age. Other strategies include selective targeting of adolescent females with monovalent rubella vaccine or screening pregnant women and offering rubella vaccine following delivery to those found to have no immunity to the disease.

In developing countries with continued high transmission rates of rubella among children, very few women of childbearing age are susceptible to the disease, and rates of CRS may be too low to warrant large-scale rubella immunization efforts. However, as an increasing number of developing countries are sustaining measles vaccine coverage at over 85%, there is a need to investigate the burden of CRS in developing countries and the cost-benefit of introducing rubella immunization.

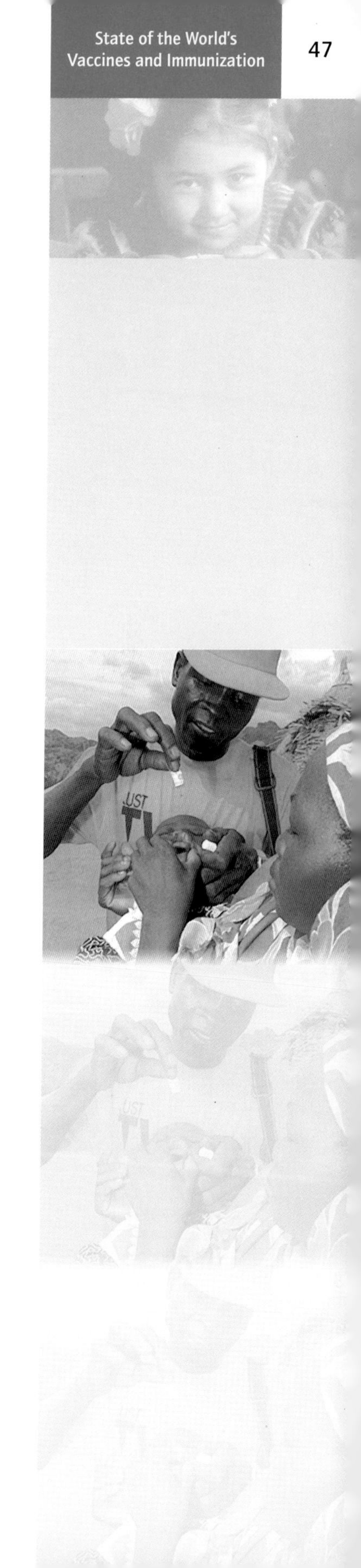

2. Eradication or elimination of vaccine-preventable diseases

- Polio
- Measles
- Neonatal tetanus

Efforts are currently under way to eradicate or eliminate three vaccine-preventable diseases – polio, measles, and maternal and neonatal tetanus – which have caused millions of deaths and immense human suffering throughout history.

The global initiative to eradicate **polio** – spearheaded by WHO, Rotary International, CDC and UNICEF – was launched by the World Health Assembly in 1988, and global certification of polio eradication is targeted for 2005. In the meantime, three WHO regions encompassing more than half the world's countries and people have been certified polio-free: the Americas (in 1994), the Western Pacific Region (including China) in 2000, and most recently the European Region in June 2002 (see Fig.12 p. 48). Since the launch of the initiative, the number of cases of polio paralysis has been dramatically reduced from an estimated 350 000 in 1988 in 125 countries to only 483 reported cases in 2001 in 10 countries.

Global targets have also been set for a major reduction in **measles** deaths worldwide and for the elimination of the disease in several large geographical areas. In 2000, measles killed 777 000 children, mainly in developing countries. The following year, a global strategic plan was drawn up by WHO, UNICEF, CDC and other global experts, in an effort to halve measles deaths worldwide by 2005 and to help efforts to eliminate the disease in areas where targets already existed. In 2005, a global consultation will review progress and assess the feasibility and desirability of an eradication initiative.

Meanwhile, efforts are continuing in order to eliminate **neonatal tetanus**, which in 2001 killed an estimated 200 000 children during their first month of life. In 1989, the World Health Assembly called for the elimination of the disease by 1995. Although this target has not yet been achieved, 104 of 161 developing countries have succeeded in eliminating the disease. In 1999, WHO, UNICEF and UNFPA set a joint target for the elimination of neonatal tetanus (a proxy indicator for maternal tetanus elimination) by 2005. To achieve global elimination of the disease, the incidence must be reduced to less than one case for every 1000 live births – not just nationwide but in every district throughout the world. The elimination initiative is supported by a partnership including national governments, UNICEF, WHO, UNFPA, CDC, PATH, Basics, Save the Children and other agencies.

Figure 12: **Polio – the last child**

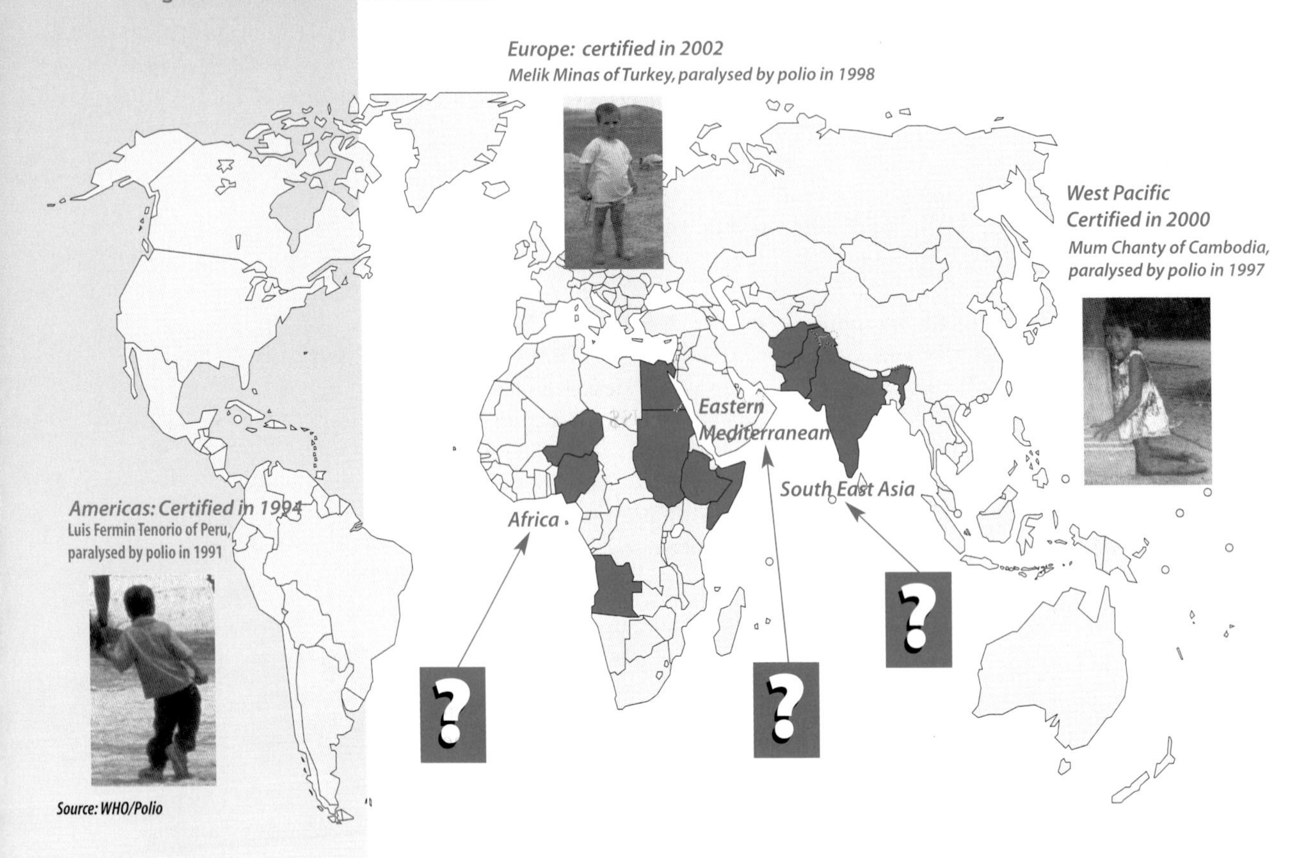

Source: WHO/Polio

Polio

With polio reduced to its lowest level in history, the race is on to immunize every child in the remaining 10 countries where poliovirus is still circulating – and to ensure that the virus is not reintroduced into any countries, especially those where the disease was, until recently, endemic. At the end of 2001, there were continued high transmission rates in the worst-affected areas: northern India, Afghanistan/Pakistan, and Nigeria/Niger. Elsewhere, the disease was still occurring, at low levels, in Angola, Egypt, Ethiopia, Somalia and Sudan.

In India, which in 2001 accounted for more than half of all remaining cases worldwide, about 40% of cases occurred in four districts in the state of Uttar Pradesh in northern India. To increase immunization coverage throughout India, nationwide campaigns have been carried out on an unprecedented scale. These have targeted every child once a month for four months in a row, followed by house-to-house campaigns in states with high transmission rates, including Uttar Pradesh, to close in on the remaining traces of the virus.

Among the countries where polio transmission is believed to have stopped are two former global reservoirs – Bangladesh and the Democratic Republic of Congo – where wild poliovirus has not been isolated for well over a year. In the Democratic Republic of Congo, despite ongoing conflict, over 11 million children were immunized in 2001 during national immunization days and surveillance was rapidly improved. As a result, the number of confirmed cases was reduced from 603 to zero within 12 months.

In 2001, over 575 million children under five years were vaccinated against polio in 94 countries around the world in the global push to eradicate the disease. The aim is to halt transmission worldwide by the end of 2002, to ensure that the world can be certified polio-free in 2005, which is only achieved three years after the last case has been identified.

In 2001, over 575 million children under five years were vaccinated against polio in 94 countries around the world in the global push to eradicate the disease

The greatest threat to the polio eradication initiative today is the lack of funding. Of the US$ 1 billion needed between 2002 and 2005, only US$ 725 million has been secured so far. Also critical is the need to secure access to children in countries affected by war and civil unrest, and to sustain political commitment at the highest level in disease-endemic and high-risk countries to ensure high quality surveillance and blanket coverage with polio vaccine. To prevent the resurgence of polio in recently endemic countries, intensified national immunization days and mop-up campaigns will be needed in the remaining polio-endemic countries until at least 2004–2005.

With so few cases remaining, the international effort has moved into the final phase – closing in on remaining polio-infected areas – while at the same time turning attention to the three areas which are critical to realizing the benefits of the polio eradication initiative: the certification process, adequately containing the remaining stocks of the virus in secure laboratories and the development of post-certification immunization policy.

Surveillance has now reached certification standard in almost all countries, guiding the immunization campaigns and verifying that countries have no more polio cases, so that regional and global certification commissions have the information needed to certify the world polio-free. The criteria for certification include an excellent standard of surveillance, as well as the appropriate containment of laboratory stocks of wild poliovirus worldwide.

Smallpox eradication taught the world a harsh lesson about the need to be as vigilant about containment of laboratory stocks of the virus as about stopping its transmission in the community. Although the last indigenous case of smallpox occurred in 1977 in Somalia, a smallpox death occurred in 1978 following an accidental release of the virus in a laboratory in Birmingham, England.

In 1999, the World Health Assembly unanimously endorsed a global plan of action for containment of polioviruses. From 2001 to 2005 all countries are required: to keep a complete inventory of all stocks of either infectious or potentially infectious virus-containing materials; to destroy non-essential stocks of wild poliovirus; and to store remaining stocks of scientific value in approved secure laboratories. One year after the last wild virus is identified, all remaining stocks must be placed in appropriate containment conditions.

WHO is overseeing an extensive programme of work which will inform post-certification polio immunization policy. Future policy options will be based on an evaluation of the risks of the reintroduction or re-emergence of polio following global certification. Known risks include those arising from the OPV, and include vaccine-associated polio paralysis, outbreaks due to circulating vaccine-derived polioviruses and immunodeficient individuals who are long-term excretors of vaccine-derived polioviruses. Episodes of circulating vaccine-derived poliovirus cases occurred in the Dominican Republic and Haiti in 2000-2001 and in the Philippines in 2001. The impact of long-term excretors who might re-seed an increasingly susceptible population in the post-immunization era is also being studied, though only 12 such individuals have been identified to date and only two of them continue to shed poliovirus.

As part of contingency planning for the post-certification era, a stockpile of polio vaccines (both oral and inactivated polio vaccines), and production capacity for these vaccines under appropriate containment conditions, will have to be maintained after vaccination stops in order to guard against any accidental or deliberate release of the vaccine. Although the threat of an intentional release of polio is low compared with either smallpox or anthrax, an emergency response plan will need to be in place if and when the use of OPV is discontinued.

The polio eradication initiative has united a wide range of coalition partners, including private foundations, development banks, donor governments, the European Commission, humanitarian and nongovernmental organizations, the corporate sector and millions of volunteers in developing countries. Since 1985, Rotary International – a prime mover in the international coalition – has committed US$ 500 million to the eradication efforts and provided volunteers in countries throughout the world. Almost two billion children have been vaccinated against polio in nationwide immunization campaigns. In 2001 alone, one-tenth of the global population was immunized.

In many countries, the polio eradication initiative has also helped strengthen immunization systems and health infrastructure. Other tangible benefits include a global

Rotary International

As the world's largest humanitarian service organizations with 1.2 million members, Rotary International is the lead private sector contributor and volunteer arm of the Global Polio Eradication Initiative. Rotary's commitment to polio eradication has its roots in 1979 with a five-year pilot immunization programme in the Philippines. Inspired by its success, in 1985 Rotary created PolioPlus – a programme to immunize all children against polio by Rotary's 100th anniversary in 2005. To date, Rotary has committed more than US$ 493 million to the protection of more than two billion children in 122 countries.

In addition, Rotary's Polio Eradication Advocacy Task Force has played a major role in decisions by donor governments to contribute over US$ 1.5 billion to the effort. This year, in an effort to help close the remaining funding gap, Rotary is embarking on its second membership fundraising drive, entitled Fulfilling Our Promise: Eradicate Polio, with the goal of raising an additional US$ 80 million for polio eradication. Rotary and the United Nations Foundation (UNF) are also collaborating in a joint appeal for funding from private corporations, foundations and philanthropists to help secure urgently needed funds by the end of 2002.

Besides raising funds to eradicate polio, over one million men and women of Rotary have volunteered their time and personal resources to help immunize children during National Immunization Days throughout the world. This extraordinary mobilization has resulted in a highly motivated and trained volunteer base. Rotary's contribution proves that civil society has a powerful role to play in public health initiatives.

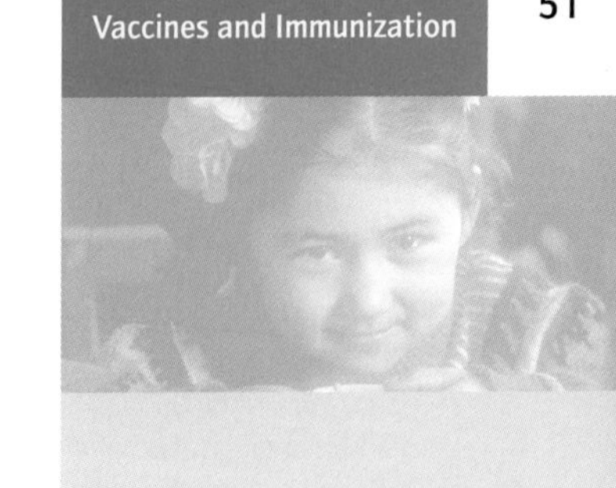

laboratory and surveillance network that can be used for other diseases, a vast human resources network trained in immunization planning and delivery, as well as a vaccine cold chain, transport and communications equipment, much of which has been replaced or refurbished with polio eradication funding. In addition, interagency coordinating committees which were established in countries to coordinate the work of the polio eradication partners under the aegis of the Ministry of Health, are now being used to help coordinate the broader immunization agenda, including the GAVI initiatives (see Box page 18).

Meanwhile, this eradication initiative has pioneered new ways of working, including: operating through a broad range of partners and mobilizing millions of volunteers to raise funds; helping to organize national immunization days; and motivating parents to bring their children to be immunized. In addition to the humanitarian benefits involved, the savings on vaccine and treatment costs following certification could potentially be as high as US$ 1.5 billion a year, which could be used to tackle other major public health problems.

Measles

Measles kills more children today than any other vaccine-preventable disease, mainly in developing countries. In 2001, there were an estimated 30–40 million cases of measles worldwide and 777 000 deaths, over one-third of all vaccine-preventable childhood deaths. Measles is one of the most contagious diseases known to man and often occurs in explosive epidemics. This disease can also lead to lifelong disabilities – including brain damage, blindness and deafness – due to encephalitis. In the developed world, where measles vaccine is widely available, serious complications and measles deaths are rare.

Throughout the 1990s, reported global routine immunization coverage with measles vaccine was only about 70%. Measles vaccine is given at least six months after the initial series of immunizations, and drop-out rates are high in some countries. In 2001, in 16 countries, most of them in Africa, less than half of children under one year old were immunized against measles. Yet measles vaccine costs only about US$ 0.26 a dose (including the cost of safe injection equipment) and is one of the most cost-effective of all health interventions.

Measles outbreak in UK following vaccine controversy

In the UK, where measles was a disappearing disease until recently, an unfounded controversy about the safety of the combined measles, mumps and rubella vaccine (MMR) has contributed to a fall in immunization rates in some areas and an outbreak of the disease. In London, where MMR coverage among two-year-olds is now 73% (compared to 84% nationwide) an outbreak occurred in 2001–2 involving 90 cases, almost half of them children aged 1–4 years.

The controversy followed the publication of a paper in a leading medical journal in 1998, which suggested there was a link between the live measles virus in the vaccine and the development of autism and inflammatory bowel disease. The theory was seized upon by the anti-vaccine lobby and widely reported in the media, provoking strong public reaction against the vaccine.

Subsequent studies have shown that the theory was not supported by any scientific evidence. WHO has firmly endorsed the use of MMR, underlining its convincing record of safety and efficacy. However, some parents, lulled into a sense of security by the low level of measles incidence in the UK, have shunned the MMR vaccine and requested changing to the use of three separate vaccines instead. The UK government, acting on independent scientific advice, has confirmed that it will continue to use MMR vaccine, pointing out that experience in the UK and elsewhere has shown that the use of separate vaccines would put children unnecessarily at risk between vaccines, increase the overall number of injections needed and lead to higher drop-out rates, thereby increasing the risk of a resurgence of all three diseases.

Where immunization coverage is high and the disease is rare, the balance between the risks and benefits of vaccination may be less clear-cut. It can be difficult to convince parents that the risk of vaccine-related adverse events is exceedingly small compared with that of contracting the disease itself. Transmitting clear evidence-based information to the public remains a significant challenge for public health officials at a time when public trust for officialdom is low, and when people are exposed to conflicting information on vaccines – not all of which is evidence-based.

Measles elimination in southern Africa

From 1996, seven countries in southern Africa, with a total population of about 70 million people, implemented measles elimination strategies. In addition to routine measles immunization at nine months of age, nationwide catch-up campaigns among children from nine months to 14 years were held, and follow-up campaigns were conducted every 3–4 years among children aged 9–59 months. In addition, there was the establishment of case-based measles surveillance with serologic diagnostic confirmation.

Reported measles cases declined from 60 000 in 1996 to 117 laboratory-confirmed measles cases in 2000. Reported measles deaths declined from 166 in 1996 to zero in 2000. This illustrates that a dramatic reduction in measles mortality and morbidity can be achieved in very low-income countries, even when the prevalence of HIV/AIDS is extremely high.

Source: R. Beillik et al, *The Lancet* 2002, 359:1564-68

Vaccination coverage for measles needs to be above 90% to stop transmission of the virus – not only because measles is so contagious, but also because up to 15% of those vaccinated at nine months fail to develop immunity. However, many countries have made dramatic progress in controlling measles. The disease is currently occurring at a very low level or has been interrupted in the Americas, Australia, Mongolia, New Zealand, the Pacific Island States, the Philippines, and in some countries in the Eastern Mediterranean Region and Europe. In some countries in Eastern Europe, an increase in immunization coverage has resulted in a dramatic decline in the number of measles cases (see Figure 13). In the Americas, which set a goal of interrupting indigenous measles transmission by the end of 2000, measles cases fell from around 250 000 cases in 1990 to 537 confirmed measles cases in 2001, the lowest number ever recorded. Key factors in this achievement included: the countries' commitment to the PAHO-recommended strategy of "catch-up, keep-up and follow-up" immunization; a determined policy of house-to-house visits in high-risk areas to ensure that every child was vaccinated; and consistent use of house-to-house monitoring during immunization campaigns to ensure that coverage targets were reached in every municipality – regardless of the quality of immunization records or the accuracy of population data.

Against all the odds, other low-income countries have also succeeded in increasing measles vaccine coverage. In Cambodia, measles vaccination coverage rates nearly doubled from just 34% in 1990 to 59% in 2001. Elsewhere, in Mozambique, coverage increased from 59% in 1990 to 92% in 2001. In southern Africa, the use of routine immunization together with immunization campaigns has had a remarkable impact on the incidence of measles cases and deaths (see Box).

The challenge now is to bring about similar dramatic improvements in coverage, and maintain them, in the countries worst affected. To achieve this, WHO, UNICEF, CDC, developing country health experts and other partners, are spearheading a major five-year effort to halve measles deaths worldwide by 2005 and interrupt indigenous measles transmission in large geographical areas.

The plan is to boost routine coverage with supplementary campaigns in an effort to achieve near blanket coverage (over 90%) and halt transmission of the virus. Each country is to draw up a three to five-year plan based on four key strategies:

- To increase routine coverage with at least one dose of measles vaccine to at least 90% of infants aged nine months.
- To provide a second opportunity for measles vaccination – either through a supplemental campaign or a routine second dose – to increase the chances that everyone gets at least one dose. The aim is to vaccinate any children who may have slipped through the net the first time round and to also provide a second opportunity for the 15% of children who may not have developed a protective immune response when vaccinated the first time.
- To establish an effective system to monitor coverage and maintain measles surveillance.
- To improve the management of complicated measles cases.

WHO and UNICEF have urged all countries to implement their plans for universal measles vaccine coverage immediately, whatever their current measles status, in a global effort to reduce measles deaths. Countries or regions with elimination plans already in place – such as the Americas, Europe and the Eastern Mediterranean – are also encouraged to work within this framework. Vitamin A is also being provided together with immunization, where needed.

Figure 13: **Reported measles cases and coverage with MCV* – Eastern European Region 1971–2000**

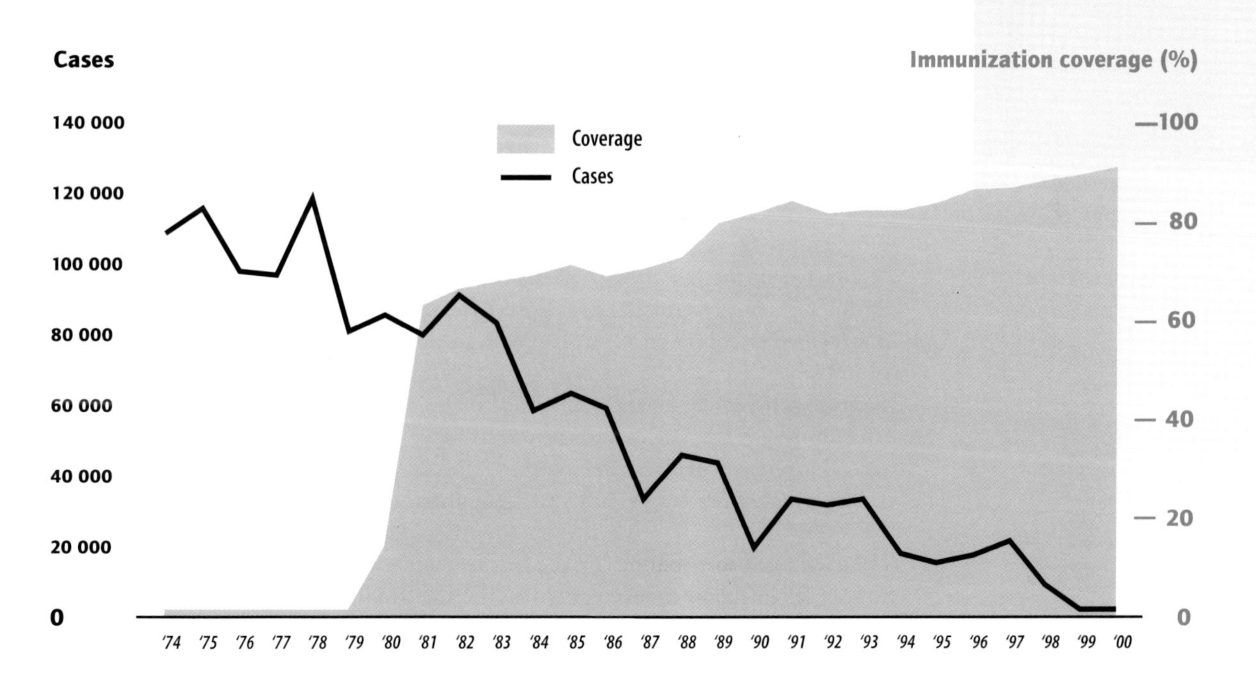

Source: WHO
** MCV Measles-containing vaccine*

Figure 14: **Maternal and neonatal tetanus elimination status as of July 2002**

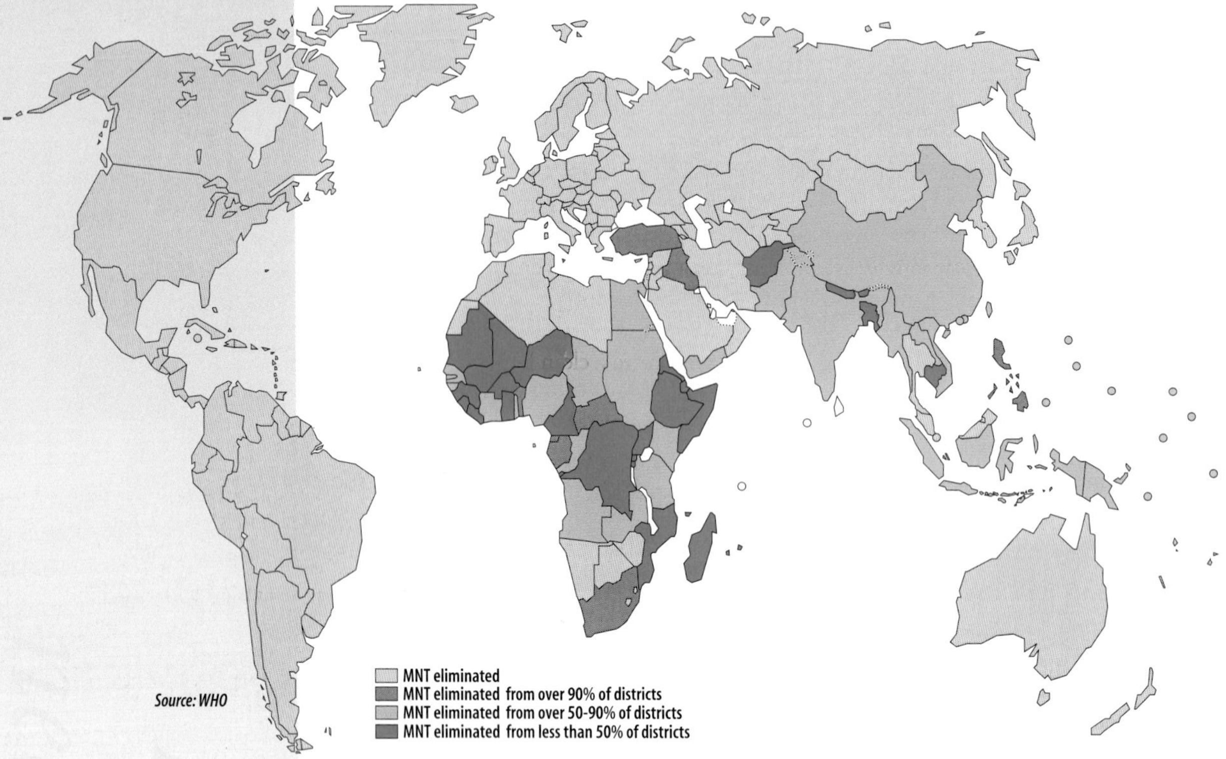

MNT eliminated
MNT eliminated from over 90% of districts
MNT eliminated from over 50-90% of districts
MNT eliminated from less than 50% of districts

Source: WHO

Maternal and neonatal tetanus

Although neonatal tetanus was eliminated in the developed world more than half a century ago, the disease still claims the lives of 200 000 babies each year in developing countries. Accelerated efforts to eliminate the disease globally by 2005 have focused attention on a disease now almost exclusively linked to poverty.

Neonatal tetanus remains a public health problem in 57 countries. Of these, 27 countries – 18 in Africa and the rest in South-East Asia and the Middle East – account for 90% of all cases. However, in Malawi, Namibia and Zimbabwe, for example, the disease has virtually been eliminated (see Fig. 14).

Neonatal tetanus strikes during the first few weeks of life when babies are most vulnerable. Infection usually starts because the umbilical cord stump has been exposed to dirt containing tetanus spores, most often through dirty hands, use of a soiled implement to cut the cord, or the application of contaminated materials (such as cow dung) to the umbilical stump. Many deaths go unrecorded, with neither the birth nor the death being officially registered.

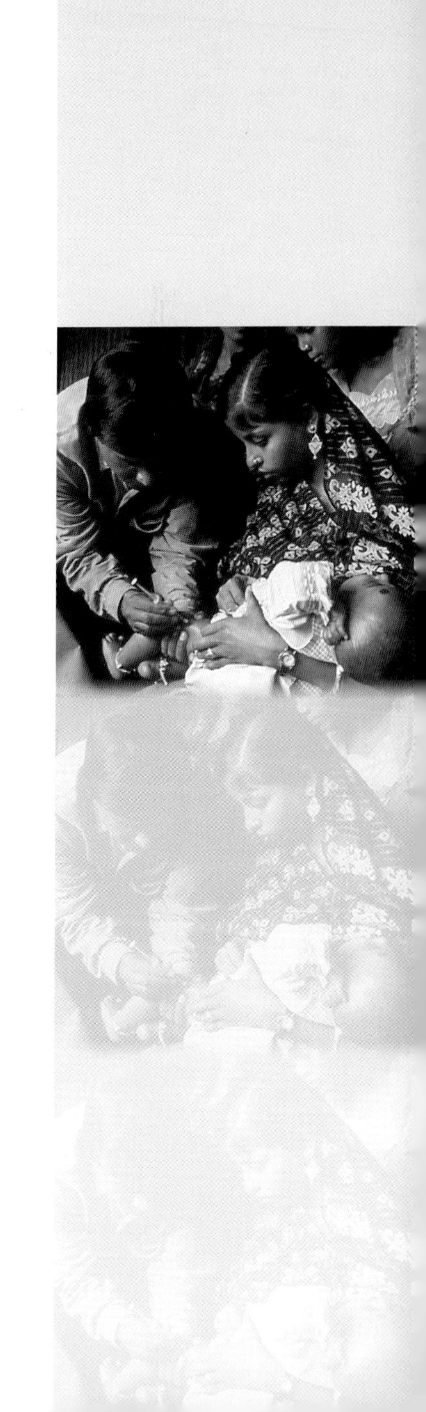

The disease has been eliminated in over 100 developing countries by ensuring that at least 90% of women in high-risk areas are fully immunized with TT during pregnancy and that they have access to a safe birth. Elimination relies on good surveillance to identify and target high-risk areas, educational strategies, immunization campaigns and door-to-door immunization.

The aim is to protect women against tetanus infection throughout their childbearing years. This ensures that they are protected against maternal tetanus – which accounts for 30 000 deaths a year worldwide – and that they can pass this immunity to their unborn child. Maternal antibodies protect newborn babies against tetanus during the first two months of life, up to the age when they themselves can be immunized with DTP vaccine. Elimination of neonatal tetanus worldwide would lead to an estimated 10–25 % reduction in infant mortality from all causes.

In Bangladesh, where most women still have no access to a clean birth or a skilled birth attendant, death rates from neonatal tetanus were reduced by over 90% between 1986 and 1998. The Bangladesh government, supported by partners including WHO, UNICEF and USAID, orchestrated nationwide immunization campaigns to immunize all women of childbearing age with TT. Thousands of vaccinators were trained and deployed throughout the country to ensure that women were reached, even those in the most remote areas. As a result, immunization coverage leapt from 5% in 1986 to 86% by 1998. Over the same period, death rates for neonatal tetanus fell dramatically from 41 deaths for every 1000 live births to only four.

In Indonesia, progress has been equally remarkable, with neonatal tetanus incidence declining from more than 20 cases per 1000 live births to less than one per 1000 live births nationwide, as immunization coverage of pregnant women with TT rose to nearly 80% in 2000. Only 63 out of 300 districts have yet to achieve the elimination target of less than one case per 1000 live births.

Tetanus toxoid is one of the cheapest, safest and most effective vaccines. It costs about US$ 1.20 on average to protect both mother and child against tetanus infection – a sum that includes the purchase and delivery cost of the vaccine and safe injection equipment as well as efforts to promote safe births.

Yet, even today, less than one in three women of childbearing age have been immunized in some of the poorest countries. In countries where over half of all districts are high-risk areas for neonatal tetanus, infrastructure is often poor, overall immunization coverage is low, or there may be severe logistical constraints, including war or civil unrest.

Because spores of the bacterium that causes the disease *(Clostridium tetani)* survive in the environment even without human contact, tetanus can never be eradicated. Routine immunization and disease surveillance will have to continue, together with efforts to promote safe births, even when the elimination target has been reached.

3. Priority new vaccines

- HIV/AIDS
- Malaria
- Tuberculosis (TB)
- Pneumococcal disease
- Meningococcal disease
- Rotavirus diarrhoea

Of all the vaccines currently under development, the three most urgently needed today are vaccines to prevent HIV/AIDS, tuberculosis and malaria. Together, these diseases account for over five million deaths a year, about half of all deaths from infectious diseases. There is no effective vaccine against HIV/AIDS or malaria. And while the existing TB vaccine (BCG) offers limited protection against childhood forms of the disease, immunity is believed to wane during adolescence.

In developing countries, where these diseases are most prevalent, the social and economic consequences have been disastrous. In many of the worst-affected countries, life expectancy has fallen by up to 20 years, the poor have been driven deeper into poverty, national income has declined and development has been set back.

Although a number of low-cost interventions exist to either prevent or treat all three diseases, some of the least-developed countries do not have the resources or policies needed to make these widely available on a sustainable basis. From 2002, the Global Fund to fight AIDS, Tuberculosis and Malaria is making funds available to some of the least-developed countries for the supply of low-cost interventions. These include bednets to prevent malaria, DOTS (Directly Observed Treatment Short Course) to treat TB, and drugs to prevent mother-to-child transmission of HIV.

Safe and cost-effective vaccines against each of these diseases would prevent millions of deaths every year and help countries in their social and economic recovery. They would also help lower the increasing threat of antimicrobial resistance to existing treatments in the worst-affected countries. However, current levels of investment in vaccine R&D do not reflect the magnitude of the threat which these diseases pose to this and future generations. Although HIV/AIDS and TB also occur in the developed countries (albeit at a much lower level) and a malaria vaccine would be useful for the expanding travellers' market, most of the vaccine sales would be in the developing world. The uncertain demand for new vaccines in developing countries has deterred vaccine manufacturers from long-term investment in the development of vaccines against HIV/AIDS, malaria and TB, which remain three of the most scientifically challenging vaccines ever investigated.

While vaccine R&D for some diseases is slowed by the low or uncertain demand for new vaccines in developing countries, the introduction of other vaccines to these countries is stalled despite the fact that they have long been licensed and widely introduced in the developed countries. The problem is that new vaccines against high-burden diseases that occur worldwide are often tailored to the form of the disease that occurs mainly in the developed world and are not appropriate for use in developing countries.

A new pneumococcal conjugate vaccine, for example, was licensed in 2000 in the United States, where it is now used to immunize infants against pneumococcal disease. However, the vaccine does not include the key serotypes of the bacterium needed to protect children in developing countries. Similarly, a new meningitis vaccine licensed in 1999 protects against serogroup C meningococcal meningitis, the form of the disease that occurs mainly in the developed countries, but not serogroup A meningococcal disease, which occurs in explosive epidemics in sub-Saharan Africa, often with heavy loss of life.

Today, new initiatives are under way to provide market incentives for the R&D of priority new vaccines for developing countries and to fast track their introduction as soon as possible after they come onto the market, instead of 10–20 years later. These include a GAVI initiative to establish detailed plans for the accelerated introduction of a rotavirus vaccine and a new pneumococcal vaccine tailored to the needs of developing countries. What is novel about this approach is that the plan is being drawn up while the vaccine trials are still under way instead of waiting for their completion. Another innovative approach is the Meningitis Vaccine Project, a partnership spearheaded by WHO and PATH which aims to accelerate the introduction of a safe and affordable vaccine against serogroup A meningococcal disease for use in developing countries.

HIV/AIDS

Disease burden

An estimated 40 million people are today living with HIV/AIDS and about 20 million people have died over the past two decades. Every day, 15 000 people, mainly young adults, become infected with HIV. Life expectancy and child survival rates have plummeted in some of the worst-affected countries.

An estimated 40 million people are today living with HIV/AIDS and about 20 million people have died over the past two decades. Every day, 15 000 people, mainly young adults, become infected with HIV

More than 95% of HIV infections are in developing countries, two-thirds of them in sub-Saharan Africa, where over 28 million people are living with HIV. While infection rates are lower in Asia and the Pacific, where over 7 million are infected, there is a risk that localized epidemics involving mainly high-risk groups could spark off major epidemics in some of the world's most populous countries.

The disease is having a major impact on social and economic development. Poverty is increasing in many countries as households lose one or more breadwinners to AIDS. And both public services and private companies are reeling from the impact of HIV-related sickness and deaths among their workforce.

In June 2001, the United Nations General Assembly declared HIV/AIDS to be "a global emergency." Member States agreed to meet new targets for HIV

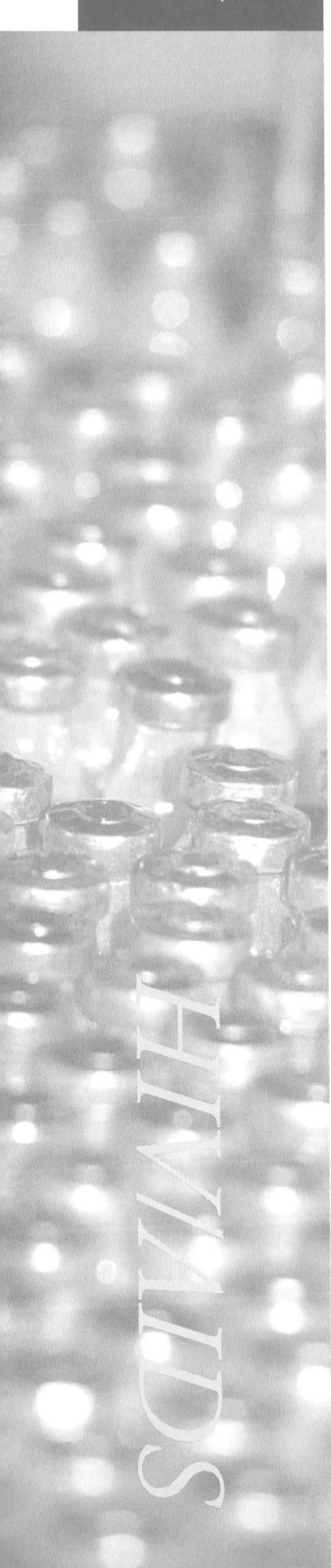

prevention and care. These included a 25% reduction in infection rates among 15–24 year olds in the worst-affected countries by 2005 (and globally by 2010) and a 20% reduction in the number of infants infected with HIV by 2005 (and by 50% by 2010).

UNAIDS and co-sponsors/partners have urged countries to implement a comprehensive package of strategies for prevention and care, including:

- access to affordable condoms
- prompt treatment of other sexually transmitted infections (which increase the risk of infection with HIV)
- access to voluntary HIV testing and counselling
- prevention of mother-to-child transmission
- promotion of advice and support to reduce HIV infection among intravenous drug users
- sexual health education in schools and the community
- improved access to care, support and treatment, including sustainable access to affordable supplies of medicines and diagnostics.

While effective HIV care and prevention strategies, together with strong political commitment, have helped reverse the tide of HIV in some countries – notably Senegal, Thailand and Uganda – a vaccine is also needed to complement existing strategies.

Vaccine update

While much more basic research is still needed, a successful vaccine against HIV is believed to be scientifically feasible (see Box page 59). However, this optimism is tempered by continued under-investment in HIV vaccine development. It is estimated that approximately US$ 600 million a year is invested in HIV vaccine R&D, the majority from the US National Institutes of Health. But not enough is being spent to develop candidate vaccines based on HIV subtypes circulating in developing countries, or to strengthen vaccine evaluation sites in these countries where 95% of infections and most deaths occur.

There are at least nine HIV-1 genetic subtypes circulating in the world. Most research to date has focused on a vaccine for HIV subtype (or clade) B, which is the main subtype in the Americas, Australia, Japan and western Europe. The subtypes mainly found in sub-Saharan Africa and Asia – where the epidemic has hit hardest – are A, C, D and E and there is no assurance that a vaccine based on subtype B will be effective against these others. In addition, vaccine efficacy may vary in different populations because of genetic make-up.

The first Phase I trial of an HIV candidate vaccine was carried out in the United States in 1987. Since then, more than 30 different candidate vaccines, developed by different companies and using different technologies, have been tested in 80 Phase I and II trials – mainly in the United States and Europe, although more recently also in developing countries (Brazil, China, Cuba, Haiti, Kenya, Peru, Thailand, Trinidad and Uganda).

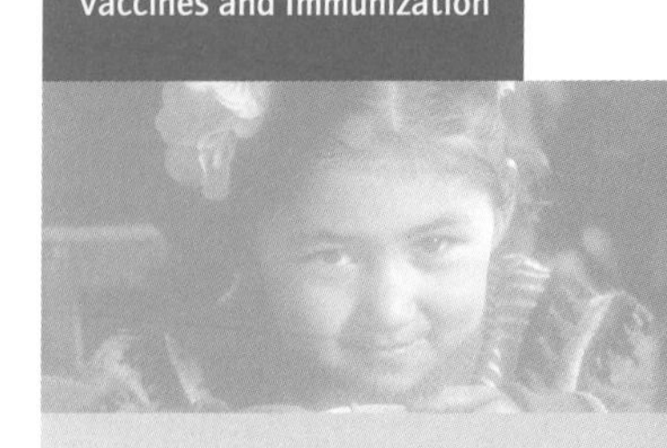

Today, 19 HIV candidate vaccines are at different levels of clinical testing in Europe, the United States and elsewhere. The first large-scale Phase III human trials of HIV vaccines are under way in the United States and Thailand. These involve 5400 volunteers in the United States, with sites in Canada and the Netherlands, and 2500 volunteers in Thailand. The trials involve the use of candidate vaccines based on gp120 (the envelope protein of HIV) corresponding to the virus types most commonly found in Europe and North America (B) and Thailand (E). Definitive results from the North American trial are expected to be available at the beginning of 2003, with results from the Thai trial a year later. While these initial trials may not result in the ideal vaccine, they may help advance the science and provide valuable information for future research efforts. The next Phase III trial, using a prime-boost combination – a canarypox-HIV recombinant vector followed by gp120 – is due to start in Thailand at the end of 2002 or beginning of 2003. Other novel candidate vaccines are being developed in the laboratory and undergoing initial Phase I/II human trials and it is expected that the best products will move to additional Phase III trials in the next 3-4 years.

In the meantime, WHO and UNAIDS are working to facilitate trials in African countries through the African AIDS Vaccine Programme (AAVP), an initiative adopted in 2001 by African Heads of State at the African Summit on HIV/AIDS, Tuberculosis and Malaria in Abuja, Nigeria. The AAVP has launched an appeal for US$ 233 million for the next seven years, to help accelerate the development and testing of a vaccine for use in Africa. Some of the funds will be used to strengthen the capacity of African research centres to conduct clinical trials of vaccine candidates.

The major manufacturers committed to HIV/AIDS vaccine R&D are Aventis Pasteur, GlaxoSmithKline, Merck & Co, and Wyeth-Lederle. Another company, VaxGen has moved products to two large-scale Phase III trials in North America and Thailand. Activities involving HIV/AIDS vaccine R&D are also supported by WHO/UNAIDS, the European Commission, United States government agencies, the UK Medical Research Council, the French Agency for Research on AIDS and the IAVI, among others. IAVI has spearheaded several projects aimed at exploring new vaccine concepts, with a focus on candidate vaccines based on HIV-1 strains prevalent in developing countries.

The scientific challenges of an HIV/AIDS vaccine

The development of a safe and effective AIDS vaccine is scientifically challenging on several fronts. An ideal vaccine must elicit immune responses capable of blocking infection by sexual, intravenous, and mother-to-child transmission. It may also need to be capable of stimulating immune responses such as antibodies that are effective in neutralizing free virus particles, as well as cellular immune responses, which destroy virus-infected cells. The induction of mucosal immunity is also being explored.

Meanwhile, the tremendous geographic diversity of HIV subtypes worldwide suggests that mixtures or "cocktails" of vaccines may be required for universal protective immunity. There is a lack of understanding of which anti-HIV immune responses are required to generate protective immunity against HIV and which components of the virus are necessary for an effective AIDS vaccine. Despite these challenges there is broad agreement within the scientific community that an effective AIDS vaccine is possible.

This optimism is based on the knowledge, firstly, that a small but growing number of people have been repeatedly exposed to HIV but have remained uninfected; they have elicited anti-HIV immune responses that could explain their resistance to infection. Secondly, there are now several candidate vaccines that have protected monkeys from infection and/or disease caused by the simian immunodeficiency virus (SIV) or the chimeric SIV/HIV (SHIV), carrying the HIV envelope; while most of these experimental vaccines did not provide complete protective immunity they were effective in significantly reducing viral loads and progression to disease in vaccinated monkeys. Thirdly, some candidate vaccines already in clinical trials have induced strong anti-HIV immune responses in human volunteers. Finally, vaccines have been successfully developed against several other viruses – measles, mumps, rubella, polio, hepatitis B and rotavirus, for example – with much less knowledge of their fundamental biology and pathogenic mechanisms than HIV.

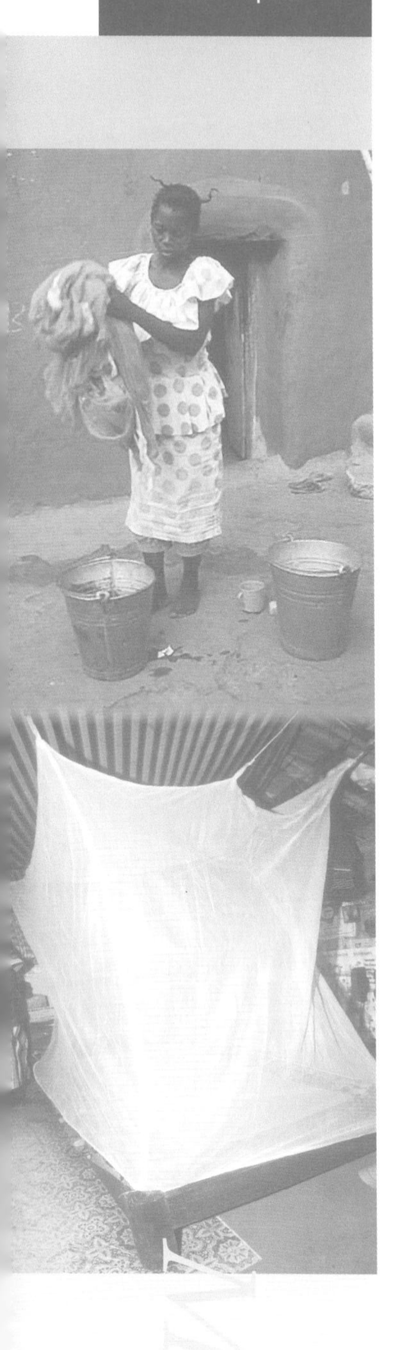

Malaria

Disease burden

Malaria is a disease that disproportionately affects the poor and is itself a major cause of poverty in the worst-affected countries. One fifth of the world's population is at risk, mainly in developing countries. There are over 300 million cases of malaria every year and over a million deaths. In sub-Saharan Africa, which accounts for over 90% of malaria deaths, almost all deaths are among children under five. In this region, malaria is responsible for one in five of all child deaths among the under-fives. Women are especially vulnerable to malaria during pregnancy when the disease can lead to life-threatening anaemia, miscarriages and the birth of premature, low birth-weight babies.

In many of the worst-affected countries, malaria parasites are showing increasing resistance to both antimalarial drugs and the most commonly-used insecticides; resistance to chloroquine, the cheapest and most widely used antimalarial drug, is widespread in Africa, and resistance to sulfadoxine-pyrimethamine, the least expensive second-line drug, is also on the increase. Moreover, mosquito populations and habitats are increasing, fuelled by changes in land and water use and by global warming. A temperature rise of only 1–2°C over the next 50 years could extend the range of malarial mosquitos to the north, further increasing the population at risk.

Malaria acts as a major brake on development, accounting for millions of days of lost productivity and missed schooling. About 60% of all malaria deaths occur among the poorest 20% of the world's population, a higher percentage than any other disease. Health economists have estimated that malaria slows economic growth in sub-Saharan African countries by over 1% a year, amounting to US$ 12 billion a year in lost earnings. In this region, malaria accounts for 40% of public health expenditure, 30–50% of hospital admissions and up to 50% of outpatient visits in high transmission areas.

In 1998, the Roll Back Malaria (RBM) partnership was established with the goal of halving the malaria burden by 2010. The RBM strategy for improved malaria control includes:

- prompt access to effective treatment
- promotion of bednets and improved vector control
- prevention and management of malaria during pregnancy
- efforts to improve the prevention of, and response to, malaria epidemics and malaria in complex emergencies.

Vaccine update

Over the past decade, there has been significant progress in malaria vaccine development, yet many valid candidate vaccines have been slow to enter clinical trials and an effective vaccine is thought be at least 10 years away. Several vaccine candidates are now being tested in Africa, Asia and the United States.

A vaccine developed in Colombia (SPf66) advanced to Phase III trials in Africa but failed to show efficacy in children under one year old, the highest risk group. Another vaccine (RTS, S/AS02) with the potential to prevent infection and/or ameliorate disease is being tested by GlaxoSmithKline and the MVI at PATH in Phase I trials in children in the Gambia. Beginning in 2002, Phase II trials of the vaccine are being conducted among children in Mozambique, which suffers from year-round malaria transmission – offering a better opportunity to evaluate vaccine performance.

This vaccine has been safely tested in adult volunteers in Belgium, the Gambia, Kenya and the United States. In the Gambia trials, the vaccine protected 70% of adults against infection (although for a few months only) making it the world's only potential malaria vaccine to have shown that level of efficacy in the field. Unlike other vaccines, a malaria vaccine even with only 50% efficacy would still be very useful in controlling the disease.

The MVI, which was established to help accelerate malaria vaccine research, is also collaborating with the International Centre for Genetic Engineering and Biotechnology (ICGEB) and the biotechnology firm Bharat Biotech International Limited, both India-based, to develop a vaccine against the malaria strain which causes nearly 65% of cases in India. In addition, the MVI has also established partnerships with biotechnology companies in the US and the UK, with the University of Oxford in the UK and with institutes in Australia to develop other candidate vaccines.

Research on malaria vaccine development is also supported by the Australian Government, Berna Biotech and Antigenics, the European Commission, the UK Medical Research Council, United States government agencies (National Institute of Allergy and Infectious Diseases, Department of Defence, USAID and CDC), VICAL (Vical, The Naked DNA Company (TM)), the Wellcome Trust, and WHO, among others. Research to date has cost about US$ 300 million.

Tuberculosis (TB)

Disease burden

An ancient scourge once thought to have been brought under control, TB is today a re-emerging disease, fuelled by the rising tide of coinfection with HIV (especially in sub-Saharan Africa) and by increasing resistance to anti-TB drugs. WHO estimates that over 17 million people are currently sick with TB.

Between 1997 and 2000 there was a 9% increase in the number of TB cases – up from 8 million to 8.7 million, of which almost 4 million were infectious ("smear positive") cases. During 2000, there were 1.7 million deaths from TB. It is estimated that almost one-third of the world's population (about 2 billion people) have latent TB infection. Of these, only about 5% will go on to develop TB at some stage in their lives. However, people coinfected with HIV and TB have an estimated 10% annual risk of developing the disease, which is a major cause of death among people with HIV/AIDS.

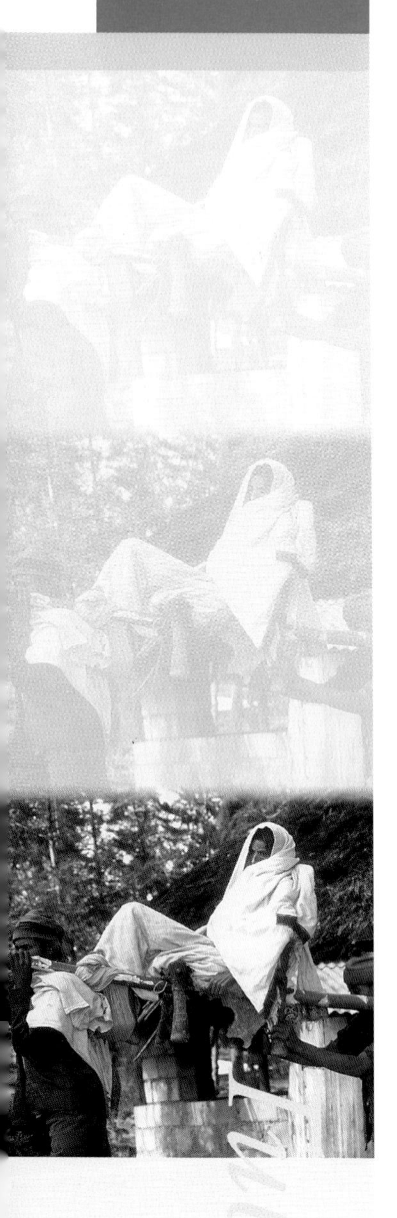

The goals set for TB control are to diagnose 70% of all infectious TB cases by 2005, and to ensure that 85% of these are successfully treated using the directly observed treatment (DOTS) strategy. Yet, these targets will not be achieved before 2013 at current rates.

In October 2001, a new US$ 9.3 billion global plan for massive expansion of TB control was issued by Stop TB – a coalition of about 120 public and private organizations – in an effort to reach the 2005 target. This called for greater investment in the R&D of new tools to combat TB, including new drugs to shorten the existing 6–8 month treatment regimen, better diagnostic tests, and a more effective vaccine with longer-lasting protection than the current vaccine, BCG. The plan also provides for a four-year investment of about US$ 1 billion to tackle the 3% of new TB cases worldwide which are now multidrug-resistant.

Vaccine update

The existing TB vaccine, BCG, developed in the early 1900s, is delivered in routine immunization programmes in most countries. It protects against miliary TB and TB meningitis in the first years of life. However, BCG is an unpredictable and imperfect vaccine. It creates an immunity that lasts at best up to the teenage years, but not for a lifetime. Its protection against adult forms of TB is variable according to: geographic location, nutritional and environmental factors, genetic make-up and type of disease. BCG is important in global immunization strategies and should be made available in global routine programmes. But a new vaccine is needed to protect against adult disease.

Genome sequencing of *M. tuberculosis* has opened the way towards a more rational approach to screening for antigens with protective capacity against TB. Promising candidates include: protein subunit vaccines; DNA vaccines expressing protective *M. tuberculosis* genes; rationally attenuated live *M. tuberculosis* vaccines; and modifications to BCG to boost its immunogenic properties. Candidate vaccines include: subunit vaccines engineered to carry protective elements from several antigens in a single molecule; prime-boost models that include BCG shots followed by DNA vaccines; and recombinant, biotechnologically "improved" BCG. If one of the candidates of this new generation of vaccines proves to be effective in humans, then a vaccine could be developed by 2012–2015.

Over the past decade, an estimated US$ 100–150 million has been spent on the development of a new TB vaccine. Key participants in this field include the Pasteur Institute (Paris), the Albert Einstein College of Medicine (New York), the Max-Planck-Institute for Infection Biology (Berlin), the University of California (Los Angeles), University of Oxford (UK) and the Statens Serum Institute (Copenhagen). Major research donors include NIH/NIAID, the European Commission, the Bill & Melinda Gates Foundation (executed by Sequella Foundation), and, importantly, a number of companies ranging from small biotechnological companies to major manufacturers.

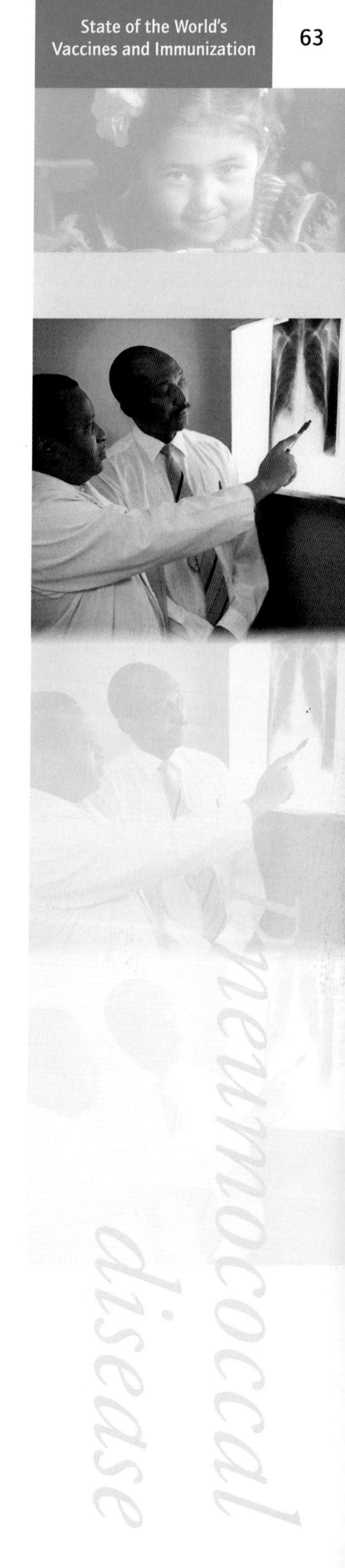

Pneumococcal disease *(Streptococcus pneumoniae)*

Disease burden

In developing countries, infection with *Streptococcus pneumoniae* accounts for most cases of bacterial pneumonia and is a major cause of death among children under five. The bacterium is also a leading cause of meningitis and middle ear infection.

Although low-cost treatment with antibiotics is available, the bacterium is increasingly resistant to first-line antimicrobial drugs and second-line drugs are often too expensive for low-income countries. An increasing number of bacteria are also resistant to multiple antibiotics, making treatment extremely difficult in resource-poor settings. Even where low-cost drugs are still effective, poor access to health care in developing countries results in high death rates. Moreover, the incidence of pneumococcal infections is being fuelled by the HIV/AIDS epidemic in some settings.

A safe and affordable vaccine against pneumococcal disease would be the most effective way of controlling pneumococcal disease and reducing the spread of drug-resistant strains of the bacterium, but the cost-effectiveness of a potential vaccine is difficult to estimate when the burden of disease is not well documented in developing countries. The problem is that the cause of the disease (as with Hib pneumonia and meningitis) is often difficult to establish. While chest x-rays are the accepted "gold standard" for diagnosis of pneumonia, variable interpretation of the results can lead to different estimates of the disease burden, and x-rays can only measure the total burden of pneumonia, not the proportion caused by pneumococcus. Meanwhile even with the best laboratory facilities, conventional microbiological techniques usually fail to determine the cause of pneumonia, especially in children.

To help establish the burden of disease in developing countries, WHO is collaborating with CDC on the development of a new protocol on disease burden, which is being pilot tested in Mozambique.

Vaccine update

One of the major challenges in developing a vaccine against *S. pneumoniae* is that the bacterium has more than 83 different serotypes. Polysaccharide vaccines which protect against the 23 serotypes which account for the most severe disease (23-valent) have been available for many years. However, these do not reliably protect children under two years, the age group most at risk.

Among the second generation pneumococcal vaccines, conjugate vaccines (modelled on the highly successful Hib conjugate vaccines) are the most advanced. A seven-valent conjugate vaccine has already been licensed by Wyeth Lederle for use in Australia, Europe, North America, and most countries in Central and South America. In trials in the United States involving about 38 000 infants, this vaccine demonstrated a high level of protection against invasive pneumococcal disease (bacteraemia and meningitis). Furthermore, in trials among 1600 infants in Finland, the vaccine was shown to protect against middle

A partnership spearheaded by WHO and PATH was launched in 2001 to put an end to the deadly meningitis epidemics that have plagued sub-Saharan Africa for more than 100 years. The Bill & Melinda Gates Foundation awarded the partnership US$ 70 million over a ten year period to develop and produce meningitis vaccines tailored for children and adults living in Africa.

ear infection caused by serotypes included in the vaccine. However, the vaccine does not include key serotypes (types one and five, for example) that are prevalent in developing countries.

To increase the protection afforded by the conjugate vaccines, candidates with as many as 11 serotypes are being developed and evaluated in clinical trials in developing countries. A nine-valent vaccine developed by Wyeth Lederle was evaluated in human trials in South Africa. The vaccine had high efficacy against invasive disease in HIV-uninfected children and moderate efficacy against invasive disease in HIV-infected children and against x-ray diagnosed pneumonia in HIV-uninfected children. The same vaccine is also being evaluated in the Gambia and an 11-valent vaccine developed by Aventis Pasteur is being tested in the Philippines, each expecting results in 2005. However, Aventis Pasteur recently announced that it will not pursue the development of this vaccine, even if the trials are successful. The company is to concentrate its efforts instead on the development of a different candidate vaccine, a protein vaccine, which is already under development but unlikely to be licensed for at least a decade.

Protein vaccines that are not serotype-specific may offer a solution to the potential limitations of conjugate vaccines, which may only be able to incorporate a limited number of serotypes. Efforts to increase the number of serotypes may complicate the conjugate vaccine production process and increase the cost of the vaccine. It is also possible that vaccine serotypes will be replaced by other non-vaccine serotypes, or transform themselves to escape the effect of the vaccine (a process known as "disease replacement").

Efficacy trials of the conjugate vaccines in Finland, South Africa and the United States, mainly supported by industry, are estimated to have cost US$ 10–30 million each. The estimated budget for the Gambia trial is more than US$ 10 million over five years and is funded through the National Institutes for Health, the Children's Vaccine Program at PATH, USAID, the Medical Research Council (UK) and WHO. It is estimated that an additional US$ 100 million will be needed to scale up the introduction of pneumococcal vaccines in developing countries.

Meningococcal meningitis

Disease burden

Meningococcal meningitis is a dreaded disease that can lead to rapid death and brain damage, especially among children. Endemic throughout the world, it can occur in explosive epidemics, especially in developing countries. Each year there are an estimated 300 000–500 000 cases of meningococcal disease and about 30 000–60 000 deaths.

Even with prompt treatment with antibiotics, 10% of patients die, usually within 24–48 hours of the onset of illness. Another 10–20% of those who survive suffer brain damage, deafness or loss of limbs.

meningococcal meningitis

Part 4 outlines some of the reasons why the world community should invest in immunization, and looks at the promising future for vaccines and immunization.

s save lives

Investing in immunization

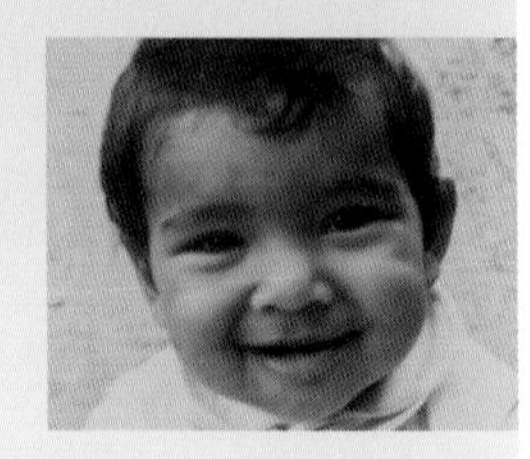

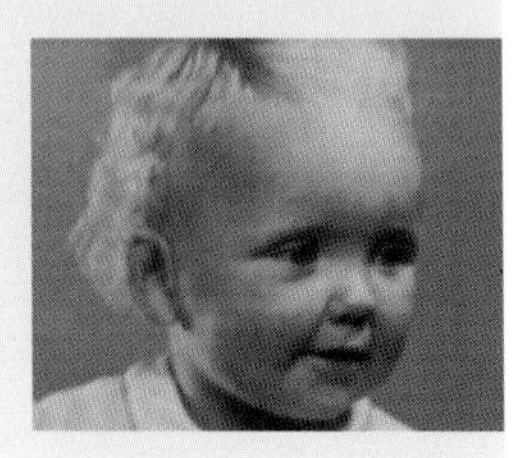

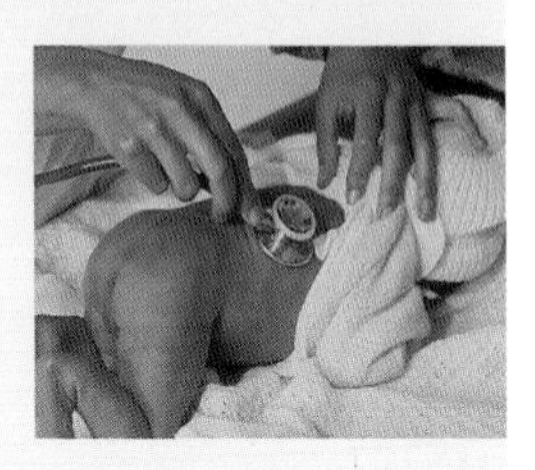

There are many reasons why the world community should invest in immunization and the reduction of infectious diseases. They include not only public health reasons but also humanitarian, economic and social reasons.

Immunization is a fundamental human right, one which governments have acknowledged by signing a succession of treaties, including the 1989 UN Convention on the Rights of the Child. The 1989 Convention adopted the definition of primary health care established by WHO Member States at the Alma Ata Conference in 1978, reconfirming the right of every child to "immunization against the major infectious diseases." But in many countries today millions of children are denied that right.

Immunization is also one of the key health interventions that can help drive economic development and poverty reduction. The poorest children are the ones least likely to be immunized and most likely to die before their fifth birthday. Those who survive and grow up in extreme poverty are the ones most likely to be trapped in a vicious cycle of malnutrition, lack of access to safe water, poor sanitation, ill health, missed schooling and unfulfilled potential – a legacy they are then likely to pass on to the next generation as well.

Immunization, together with other low-cost health interventions, can help break that vicious cycle. By preventing infectious diseases and extending life expectancy, immunization can help increase a child's capacity to learn and their capacity to earn as adults, reducing poverty and boosting the country's potential for economic growth. Recent studies have shown that the economic costs of disease in the poorest countries can run into hundreds of billions of US dollars a year in lost GNP. Immunization can help reverse that trend. In addition, by targeting infectious diseases – the main factor in differences in life expectancy between the rich and the poor – immunization can help reduce the inequalities in health.

Immunization is also one of the key health interventions that can help drive economic development and poverty reduction

Childhood vaccination is one of the most cost-effective of all health interventions – saving more lives for the money invested than almost any other health intervention available today. It costs on average US$ 25 (including delivery costs) to fully immunize a child with the six traditional EPI vaccines against diphtheria, pertussis, tetanus, polio, measles and TB, far less than the cost of treating children who succumb to vaccine-preventable diseases. In addition, the regular provision of immunization provides a vital opportunity for the delivery of other health interventions, such as supplements of vitamin A and iodine to prevent nutritional disorders.

Even in countries where the EPI package includes more expensive vaccines against hepatitis B and *Haemophilus influenzae* type b, immunization remains one of the best health investments available today. The cost-effectiveness of immunization has been further underlined by the rapid increase in antimicrobial resistance, which has made some infectious diseases increasingly difficult – and many times more expensive – to treat.

Over the past decade, events such as the re-emergence of yellow fever in Africa, the resurgence of diptheria in Eastern Europe, and the re-introduction of polio in Europe in 1996 are an ominous warning of the fragility of immunization achievements and of what can happen when immunization is neglected. Meanwhile, the benefits of immunization extend beyond those vaccinated in any country to people everywhere, and to future generations as well. The eradication of smallpox in 1979, for example, has prevented millions of deaths so far and freed up scarce resources.

Towards a brighter future

Despite years of remarkable progress during the 1980s in providing access to immunization for every child, some developing countries have been unable to increase – or in some cases even to maintain – the level of vaccination coverage that was achieved in 1990.

The Global Alliance for Vaccines and Immunization was launched in 2000 in an effort to reverse this decline, revitalize global commitment to immunization and open up access to new vaccines urgently needed in developing countries. The Alliance has made great strides over the past two years and these efforts must continue to expand. Every child fully immunized contributes to a reduction in the world's vulnerability to vaccine-preventable diseases.

Vaccines hold great promise for the future

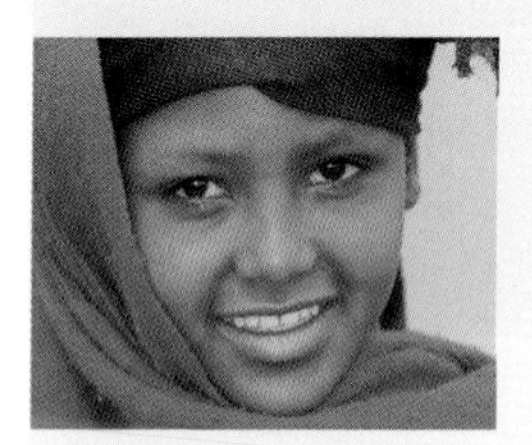

New initiatives are expected to yield vast benefits for children in low- and middle-income countries. These include a reduction in disease burden, the prospect of healthy children with the promise of a brighter future, strengthened health and immunization systems, and greater commitment among politicians and decision-makers to investing in health – and thereby investing in development.

Vaccines hold great promise for the future. New vaccines already exist that have been proven both safe and effective. The problem is that they are often unavailable where they are needed most. But there is now a greater understanding within the public sector of the vaccine production cycle and of what is needed to break this deadlock. This includes:

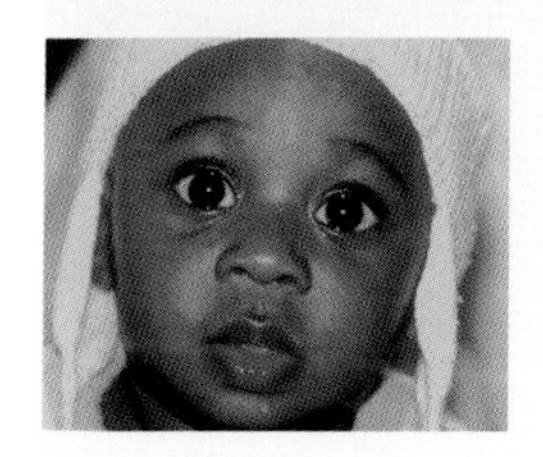

- Efforts to better understand and overcome the constraints experienced by existing manufacturers in making vaccines more affordable
- Defining the most cost-effective options for vaccine manufacture for developing countries, including increased vaccine manufacturing capacity in these countries
- Building capacity in countries to optimize the impact of vaccines and reduce wastage
- Ensuring creative and sustainable financing mechanisms and well-coordinated procurement plans
- Advocating for more equitable access to priority vaccines – both new and existing vaccines – for children who need them most.

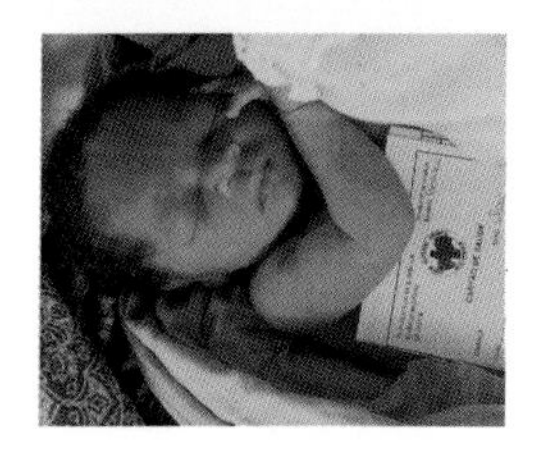

Meanwhile, on the horizon are new vaccines that promise to have a major impact on health. Some of these require laboratory-based research, while others have reached the stage where their efficacy and safety can be scientifically established through large scale trials.

It is hoped that this report has helped summarize the state of knowledge about vaccines in the world today and the great, and growing, expectations which these public health tools have created. Efforts to ensure the wider use of those vaccines already available and the discovery of new ones will largely depend on the success of new initiatives aimed at stimulating public interest and demand, fostering stronger political will, encouraging and supporting scientific research, and catalyzing and sustaining the financial resources required. END Part 4

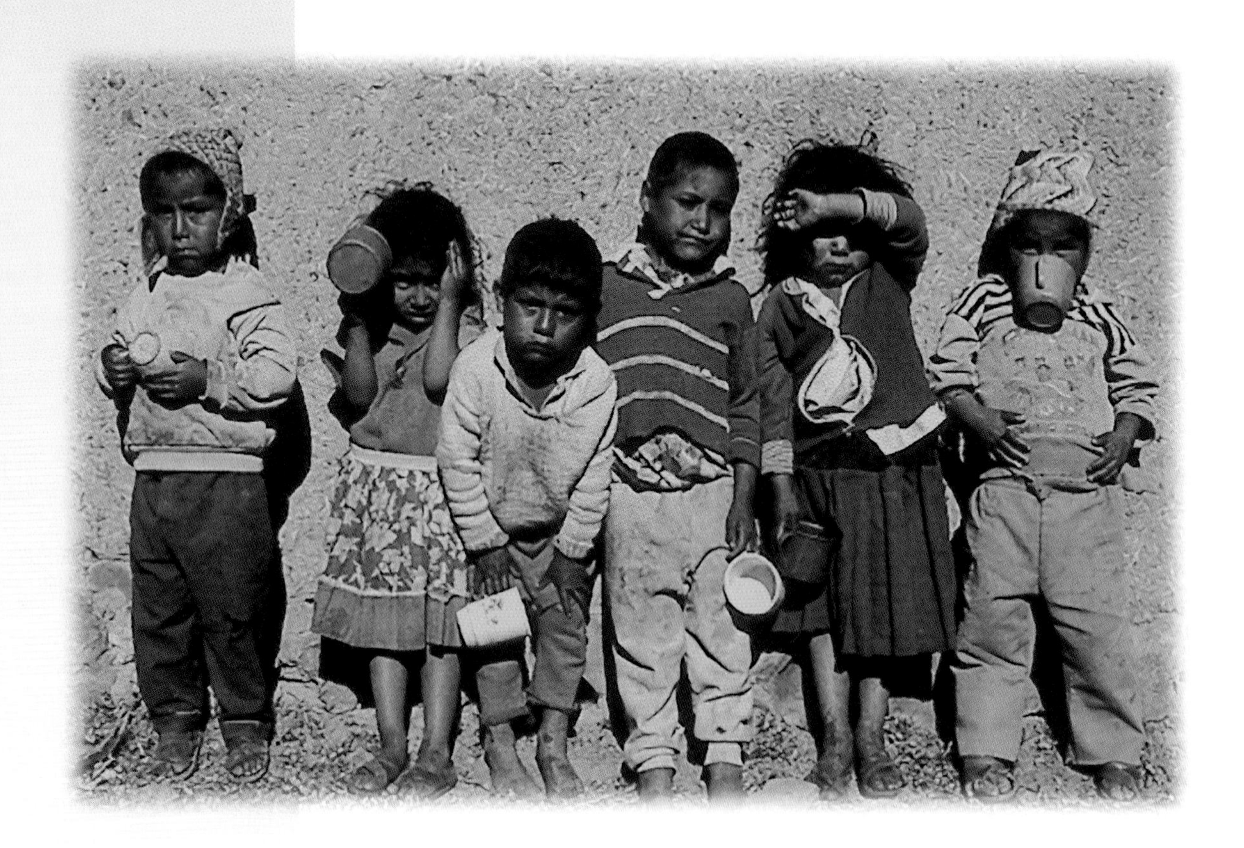

Immunization saves millions of lives each yea

Annex 1

Prequalified vaccines

Through its Department of Vaccines and Biologicals, the World Health Organization provides advice to UNICEF and other United Nations agencies on the acceptability, in principle, of vaccines considered for purchase by such agencies[1].

The system in place has been effective in promoting confidence in the quality of the vaccines shipped to countries through UN purchasing agencies and is increasingly used not only by UN agencies but also by countries seeking guidance on reliable sources of vaccines for purchase.

In recent years it has been recognized that the system should be expanded to include other vaccines that are or should be used more by countries. These include vaccines in complex multivalent combinations as well as products used for outbreaks of diseases such as cholera and meningitis.

The purpose of the assessment is to verify that the vaccines meet the specifications of the relevant UN agency, and are produced and overseen according to the principles recommended by WHO, including those for good manufacturing practices (GMP).

The aim is to ensure that vaccines used in national immunization programmes throughout the world are safe and effective and that they meet specifications for packaging and presentation.

The assessment procedure established by WHO is based on the following principles:

- Reliance on the national regulatory authority (NRA) of the country of manufacture
- General understanding of the product and presentations offered, production process, quality control methods, and relevance for the target population of available clinical data
- Assessment of production consistency through compliance with GMP specifications
- Random testing of vaccines to monitor compliance with tender specifications on a continuing basis
- Monitoring of complaints from the field.

WHO can advise UNICEF and other UN agencies whether vaccines effectively meet WHO-recommended requirements **only if the NRA of the producing country exercises independent and appropriate oversight of the vaccines in question and if the vaccines have been assessed through the procedure described above.**

However, it should be noted that other vaccines that have not gone through this process may be as safe and effective as those that have actually been assessed.

Current list of pre-qualified vaccines:
http://www.who.int/vaccines-access/vaccines/Vaccine_Quality/UN_Prequalified/UN_Prequalified_producers.htm

United Nations Prequalified Vaccines
WHO list of vaccines for purchase by UN agencies
As of August 2002

1 *The process in place at WHO to assess the acceptability of candidate vaccines for purchase was published initially in the thirty-ninth report of the WHO Expert Committee on Biological Standardization (Technical Report Series 786, Annex 1, 1989). It was further revised and replaced in 1996 by the document* Procedure for assessing the acceptability, in principle, of vaccines for purchase by United Nations agencies *WHO/VSQ/97.06).*

United Nations Prequalified Vaccines
WHO list of vaccines for purchase by UN agencies
As of August 2002

Producer	Vaccines
Aventis Pasteur, Canada	DTP, measles
Aventis Pasteur, France	BCG, DT, dT, DTP, OPV, TT, measles, MMR, Hib, yellow fever, meningococcal A + C
Biken, Japan	Measles
Bio Farma, Indonesia	DT, DTP, OPV, TT, TT filled in Uniject, measles
Biomanguinhos, Brazil	Yellow fever
Center for Genetic Engineering and Biotechnology, Cuba	Hepatitis B (recombinant)
Cheil Jedang, Korea	Hepatitis B (plasma derived)
Chiron Behring, Germany	DTP, Rabies
Chiron Behring, India	Rabies
Chiron Vaccines, Italy	DTP, MMR (measles, mumps, rubella combination), MR (measles, rubella combination), OPV, measles, Hib, DTP-Hib
CSL, Australia	DT, DTP, TT
GlaxoSmithKline, Belgium	Hepatitis B, Hib, OPV, meningococcal A + C, DTP-Hep B, DTP-Hep B to be combined with Hib (pentavalent), measles, MMR
GreenCross Vaccine Corporation, Korea	Hepatitis B (recombinant)
Human Co., Hungary	DT, TT, Td
Institut Pasteur Dakar, Senegal	Yellow fever
Japan BCG	BCG
Lucky Goldstar, Korea	Hepatitis B (recombinant)
Celltech Group plc, (formerly Medeva, U.K.)	BCG, Yellow fever
Merck and Co. Inc, USA	Hepatitis B
National Center for Infectious and Parasitic Diseases, Intervax, Bulgaria	BCG
SBL Vaccin AB, Sweden	Inactivated oral cholera
Serum Institute of India	DT, dT, DTP, TT, MR, measles
Shanta Biotechnics Private Ltd., India	Hepatitis B (recombinant)
Statens Seruminstitut, Denmark	BCG
Wyeth Lederle Vaccines and Pediatrics, USA	Hib

Annex 2

Glossary of vaccine terms

Vaccines work by mimicking a natural infection and triggering a specific immune response. They exist in a variety of formulations or compositions. Some examples are:

Aerosol vaccines: liquid vaccine atomized into a fine spray for delivery via the airways.

Canarypox: an avian virus similar to smallpox virus but because it cannot fully reproduce in humans is used as a safe vaccine-vector for other pathogens, such as HIV.

Chimeric vaccines: term used to describe two different concepts: (i) a live vaccine against pathogen A used as a vector for antigens against pathogen B, e.g. yellow fever vaccine virus genetically engineered to produce Japanese Encephalitis vaccine antigens, (ii) a vaccine composed of genetic material from more than one genetic variant or serotype of a pathogen, e.g. Human Papillomavirus.

Combination vaccines: a mixture of vaccines that target several infectious agents or pathogens at the same time, e.g. DTP, MMR.

Conjugate vaccines: formulated by chemically linking sugar chains derived from the pathogen to a protein backbone, e.g. Hib, pneumococcal vaccines.

DNA vaccines: vaccines based on genetic material; DNA acts as a vaccine 'template', injected into human tissues, which instructs human cells on the precise structure of the vaccine and engineers its synthesis. DNA vaccines against influenza, hepatitis B and HIV are in development but not yet on the market.

Envelope protein: the protein located in the outside of HIV (gp120)

Epitope-based cocktail vaccines: products which include multiple protein stretches which are believe to induce immunity (epitopes)

Infectious clone: Normally referred to a DNA molecule equivalent to the complete genome of a virus, capable of generating infectious viruses when introduced into a susceptible cell.

Live attenuated vaccines: vaccines based on genetic 'impairment' of the pathogen, which eliminates the disease-provoking qualities while maintaining the capacity to trigger an immune response, e.g. measles, polio, cholera.

Lyophilized vaccines: formulations of vaccines that have been freeze-dried during manufacture before the vial is sealed. They need reconstituting with liquid before use.

Monovalent vaccines: vaccines containing only one antigen.

Mucosal vaccines: vaccines formulated most commonly for oral or nasal delivery, e.g. oral polio vaccine.

Protein vaccines: vaccines based on one or several isolated proteins obtained from the pathogen, e.g. tetanus toxoid, or through genetic engineering, e.g. acellular pertussis.

Polysaccharide vaccines: vaccines based on sugar components derived from surface structures of the infectious agent, e.g. pneumococcal, meningococcal A/C.

Polyvalent vaccines: a mixture of vaccines targeted at different strains or subtypes of the same pathogen, e.g. seven-valent pneumococcal.

Prime boost effect: Normally a prime-boost regime implies two or more administration of the same vaccine, to increase the immune response. Prime-boost combination in HIV vaccine research also refer to the sequential administration of two different candidate vaccines to induce both humoral and cell-mediated immunity against the virus.

Recombinant vaccines: genetically engineered vaccines developed by molecular cloning that takes one or several genes from the infectious agent and expresses them in a host, e.g. hepatitis B.

Serotypes: Different immunological varieties of the same pathogens, which may not induce cross-protective immunity.

Simian immunodeficiency virus (SIV): a virus similar to human immunodeficincy virus (HIV) occurring in monkey species.

Subunit vaccines: based on isolated elements of the pathogen, e.g. protein, DNA or polysaccharide vaccines.

Whole cell vaccines: based on the entire pathogen, e.g. killed, live attenuated vaccines.

Annex 3

This table shows a typical schedule for the first 9 months of life in an African country that has endemic yellow fever. It would typically cost around US$ 5 to purchase the vaccines and another US$ 20 of indirect costs to administer them per child.

A national immunization schedule for infants in developing countries

Vaccine	Age				
	Birth	6 weeks	10 weeks	14 weeks	9 months
BCG	x				
Oral polio	x*	x	x	x	
DTP		x	x	x	
Hepatitis B◆		x	x	x	
Haemophilus influenzae type b◆		x	x	x	
Yellow fever					x**
Measles					x***

* *In endemic counties*

** *In countries where yellow fever poses a risk.*

*** *In addition, a second opportunity to receive a dose of measles vaccine should be provided for all children. This may be done either as part of the routine schedule or in a campaign.*

◆ *Only a few African countries have been able to introduce the vaccines to date*

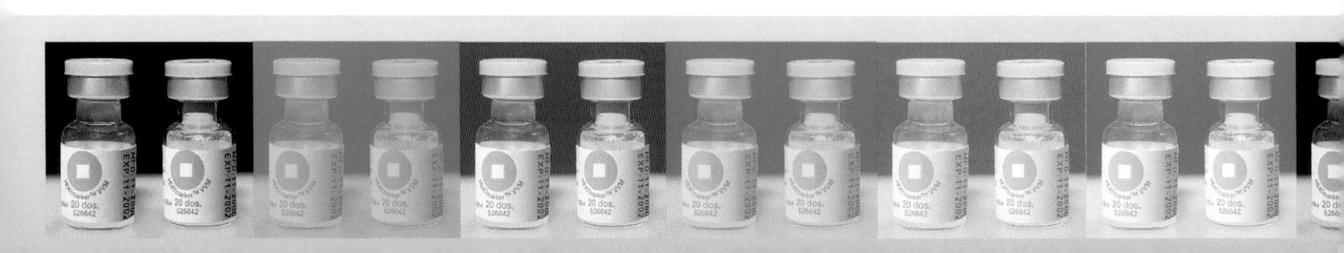

This table shows a typical infant immunization schedule for an affluent industrialized country. The cost of the vaccines would typically be around US$ 300 (more in the private sector) plus the cost of the visit to the practitioner that is highly variable both between countries and within each country. It could be as high as US$ 400 for administration of all vaccines to a child in the first five years of life. This represents a striking difference, with more antigens, more doses, more visits and at higher cost than in developing countries.

A national immunization schedule for infants in industrialized countries

Vaccine	Age							
	Birth	1 month	2 months	3 months	4 months	5 months	6 months	+1 year (5)
BCG (6)	x							x
Hepatitis B	x (1)	x			x		x	
DTP or DTaP			x		x		x	
Haemophilus influenzae type b			x	x	x			
Oral or inactivated polio			Oral/IPV	Oral/IPV	Oral		IPV	
Measles, Mumps and Rubella (MMR)								x
Pneumococcal			x		x		x	
Other vaccines (2):								
• Influenza (3)							x	
• Varicella								x
• Hepatitis A (4)								variable

(1) Given with HBIG(hepatitis B immunoglobulin) if mother is HBsAg-positive (surface-antigen positive)
(2) Only used by some countries, and frequently only for selected populations
(3) Generally only given from 6 months of age to high risk selected infants annually
(4) Generally only given to high risk selected infants in the first year of life
(5) Variable additional doses of these vaccines are scheduled as boosters during the next two decades
(6) BCG is administered in certain industrialized countries, but to widely differing ages and in varying numbers of doses.

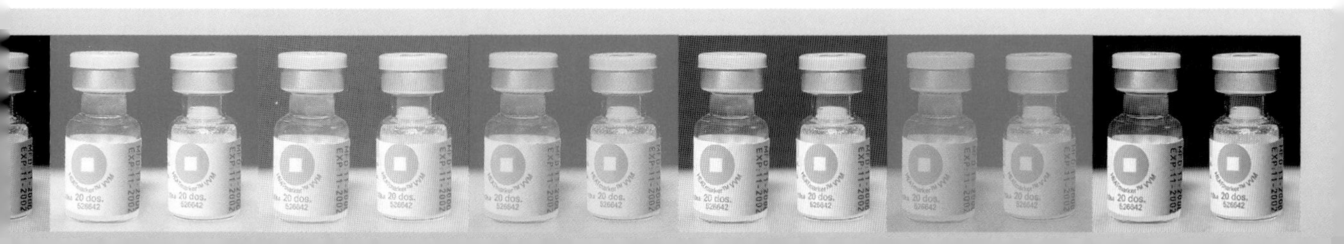

Annex 4

Statistical annex

Background:

Coverage levels with diphtheria and tetanus toxoid and pertussis vaccine (DTP) are considered one of the best indicators of health system performance, and funding agencies frequently consider immunization coverage levels when reviewing applications for financial and technical support.

In June 2000, the World Health Organization (WHO) and the United Nations Children's Fund (UNICEF) began a retrospective review of national immunization coverage for the years 1980-1999. Estimates were made for the third dose of diphtheria, tetanus toxoid and pertussis vaccine (DTP3). The review, completed in October 2001, has been continued and currently includes estimates of national immunization coverage for the years 2000 and 2001.

The estimates on immunization coverage provided in the follwing table relate to the years 1980, 1990, and 2000. A map showing DTP3 estimates for 2001 can be found on p. 96. WHO/UNICEF have produced and compiled these estimates, which have been shared with National Ministries of Health for review and comments, but are not necessarily the official estimates used by national governments.

The WHO/UNICEF review (data, methods and process):

Based on the data available, consideration of potential biases, and contributions from local experts we have attempted to determine the most likely true level of immunization coverage.

For this review we have relied on the following data:
1. Officially reported data by member states to WHO.
2. The historical database maintained by UNICEF.
3. The published literature – primarily coverage survey results and methods.
4. Unpublished surveys available from ministries of health.

Immunization coverage levels are presented as a percentage of a target population that has been vaccinated.

Country	1980					1990					2000				
	Births	BCG	DTP3	*MCV	**Pol3	Births	BCG	DTP3	*MCV	**Pol3	Births	BCG	DTP3	*MCV	**Pol3
Afghanistan	732,478		4	11	3	704,035	30	25	20	25	1,050,615	38	31	35	32
Albania	73,184					80,260	94	94	88	89	61,370	93	97	95	97
Algeria	811,573					774,599	99	89	83	89	747,517	97	92	80	90
Andorra						0					0		90	90	90
Angola	360,760					495,747	48	24	38	23	675,182	56	31	46	33
Antigua and Barbuda			54		36	0		99	89	99	0		99	99	99
Argentina	694,323	62	41	58	91	693,217	99	86	93	90	721,458	99	66	56	85
Armenia						0					36,800	97	93	92	96
Australia	227,654		33		17	253,179		95	86	72	248,819		92	92	91
Austria	88,605					91,274		90	60	90	74,045		81	75	71
Azerbaijan						0					110,871	99	99	99	99
Bahamas	5,806		36		35	6,041		87	86	86	6,182		99	93	91
Bahrain	11,574		72	45	72	14,127		94	87	94	10,824		97	98	97
Bangladesh	3,593,485					4,066,009	86	69	65	69	4,217,433	95	83	76	83
Barbados	4,347		60	41	99	3,844		91	87	90	3,342		94	91	86
Belarus			82		80	0	91	89	96	90	90,739	198	198	196	198
Belgium	119,905					121,135		93	85	95	104,637		96	83	96
Belize	5,712	65	47	21	21	6,383	86	91	86	86	6,064	95	89	96	89
Benin	179,376					221,953	92	74	79	74	263,439	94	79	68	78
Bhutan	54,857	43	6	21	4	66,952	99	96	93	96	73,753	97	92	76	98
Bolivia	210,238	30	11	13	14	238,898	65	41	53	50	265,718	95	80	79	78
Bosnia and Herzegovina	0					0					38,181	93	85	80	87
Botswana	40,715	92	71	63	46	47,810	93	92	87	90	49,021	99	97	90	97
Brazil	3,805,708	56	37	56	69	3,512,714	79	66	78	58	3,354,455	99	95	99	99
Brunei	5,907		89	73	89	6,998	91	93	99	92	6,703	99	99	99	99
Bulgaria	131,761					102,248	99	99	98	99	61,711	97	93	87	98
Burkina Faso	346,360					428,506	95	66	79	66	542,850	72	41	46	42
Burundi	190,164					261,337	96	85	74	85	277,554	84	74	75	69
Cambodia	317,024					419,150	52	38	34	39	476,021	81	59	65	62
Cameroon	395,633					488,219	76	48	56	54	548,265	80	53	62	49
Canada	368,911					391,177		88	89	88	344,409		97	96	89
Cape Verde	10,704					11,883	97	88	79	87	13,076	92	86	80	86
Central African Republic	101,112	17	13	12	13	123,561	93	82	83	82	142,881	47	29	34	31
Chad	217,075					282,462	59	20	32	20	383,189	50	28	42	29
Chile	258,341	88	85	99	77	298,298	94	99	82	97	288,264	97	97	97	98
China	20,142,244					23,681,538	99	97	98	98	19,253,606	85	85	85	90

* Measles containing vaccine (M, MR, MMR)

** 3 doses of polio vaccine (OPV or IPV)

Country	1980 Births	1980 BCG	1980 DTP3	1980 *MCV	1980 **Pol3	1990 Births	1990 BCG	1990 DTP3	1990 *MCV	1990 **Pol3	2000 Births	2000 BCG	2000 DTP3	2000 *MCV	2000 **Pol3
Colombia	889,493	45	16	13	16	961,634	95	88	82	93	980,870	86	74	75	78
Comoros	19,030					21,329	99	94	87	94	27,229	90	70	70	70
Congo	74,835					99,633	90	79	75	80	134,675	50	33	34	33
Costa Rica	70,947	80	86	60	86	83,161	92	95	90	95	90,850	92	88	82	80
Cote d´Ivoire	435,880					524,969	62	54	56	56	570,963	84	72	73	72
Croatia	0					0					54,791	99	93	93	94
Cuba	153,310	99	67	48	99	174,008	98	92	94	94	137,295	99	95	94	99
Cyprus	12,464					12,642					10,471		97	86	97
Czech Republic	0					0					88,192	98	98	97	98
Czechoslovakia	257,973					207,207	98	99	99	99	0				
Denmark	56,349					63,274		95	84	97	62,651		97	99	97
Djibouti	16,185					21,967	81	85	85	85	24,405	34	46	50	46
Dominica	0	65	63		53	0	99	96	91	98	0	99	99	99	99
Dominican Republic	196,412	12	36	30	46	203,101	70	69	96	90	199,741	90	68	88	54
DPR Korea	345,060					416,616					392,360	64	37	34	77
DR Congo	1,293,646	57		18	15	1,797,531	65	35	38	34	2,441,739	57	40	46	42
Ecuador	291,921	76	10	24	19	303,265	89	68	60	67	308,657	99	89	84	81
Egypt	1,721,269	50	57	41	67	1,776,635	89	87	86	87	1,682,999	98	98	98	98
El Salvador	167,760	56	44	45	42	154,574	75	80	98	80	166,903	99	99	97	98
Equatorial Guinea	10,033					15,516	94	77	88	75	19,833	34	32	19	32
Eritrea	107,270					134,225					147,415	98	93	88	93
Estonia	0					0					11,852	99	93	93	93
Ethiopia	1,648,126			4	3	2,216,967	64	49	38	49	2,787,897	76	56	52	57
Federated States of Micronesia	0					0					0	24	85	85	85
Fiji	20,973	95	68	32	55	20,805	99	97	84	96	20,491	98	89	85	95
Finland	65,625					64,156	91	90	97	90	53,691	99	99	96	95
France	754,410					751,130	80	95	71	85	732,010	84	98	84	97
Gabon	22,618					34,131	96	78	76	78	46,591	89	38	55	31
Gambia	31,109	85	63	69	53	41,638	98	92	86	94	50,485	97	83	85	89
Georgia	0					0	95	91	99		57,059	95	80	73	81
Germany	817,437					845,339		80	50	85	718,374		97	89	95
Ghana	518,760		7	16	7	594,909	71	58	61	57	642,082	95	84	84	83
Greece	143,003		72		90	103,043	86	54	76	96	97,452	88	88	88	87
Guatemala	299,652	36	43	23	43	346,165	62	66	68	74	404,252	97	85	88	85
Guinea	242,864					277,978	50	17	35	18	364,535	71	46	52	43
Guinea-Bissau	33,865					42,884	90	61	53	60	53,955	72	42	59	47

* Measles containing vaccine (M, MR, MMR)

** 3 doses of polio vaccine (OPV or IPV)

Country	1980					1990					2000				
	Births	BCG	DTP3	*MCV	**Pol3	Births	BCG	DTP3	*MCV	**Pol3	Births	BCG	DTP3	*MCV	**Pol3
Guyana	23,187	68	35		42	18,115	82	83	77	78	17,413	93	88	86	78
Haiti	231,099		3		8	258,353	72	41	31	40	254,434	71	43	54	43
Honduras	156,113	25	28	31	31	187,198	70	84	90	87	203,913	99	95	98	86
Hungary	154,518	99	99	99	98	124,318	99	99	99	99	91,572	99	99	99	99
Iceland	4,259					4,467		99	99	99	4,030		98	91	95
India	23,561,212		6		2	25,534,003	66	70	56	66	25,204,253	73	64	56	70
Indonesia	5,073,668	61				4,802,919	74	60	58	60	4,496,973	75	61	56	67
Iran (Islamic Republic of)	1,786,412	7	32	39	38	2,080,682	95	91	85	90	1,566,319	99	99	99	99
Iraq	534,402	76	14	9	16	685,976	96	83	80	83	812,930	93	81	90	86
Ireland	73,050		34		72	52,119	84	65	78	81	55,721	90	86	77	86
Israel	93,477	75	84	81	85	100,817		93	91	93	125,441		96	94	92
Italy	657,309					556,235		83	43	98	510,726		95	70	96
Jamaica	59,712	38	24		34	56,941	98	86	69	87	53,574	94	86	88	86
Japan	1,630,048		60	69		1,222,947	85	90	73	90	1,208,908	96	85	96	99
Jordan	97,999		30	29	32	128,254		92	87	92	166,054		91	94	94
Kazakhstan	0					0	87	80	95	85	264,939	98	97	99	97
Kenya	842,470					988,323	92	84	78	84	1,064,307	91	76	76	73
Kiribati	0					0					0	80	90	80	90
Kuwait	51,248		67	48	70	48,134		71	66	71	32,123		98	99	94
Kyrgyzstan	0					0					103,398	96	99	98	99
Lao PDR	146,649					178,579	26	18	32	26	194,863	69	53	42	57
Latvia	0					0					17,910	99	97	97	96
Lebanon	80,165					75,662		82	61	82	67,678		90	90	90
Lesotho	56,146					63,273	97	76	80	76	68,414	92	85	77	84
Liberia	90,092					86,827					157,149	79	55	52	59
Libyan Arab Jamahiriya	147,065	88	60	61	60	116,154	90	84	89	84	142,684	97	94	92	94
Lithuania	0					0					34,159	99	94	97	92
Luxembourg	4,126					4,849		90	80	90	5,445		98	91	98
Madagascar	413,771	21				536,187	67	46	47	46	685,896	72	55	55	58
Malawi	340,964		58	49	28	466,387	97	87	81	93	517,669	83	75	83	73
Malaysia	422,564	94	67		67	553,431	99	90	70	90	525,009	99	95	88	95
Maldives	6,634	7	4		4	8,564	99	94	96	94	10,649	99	97	99	97
Mali	346,354					440,107	82	42	43	42	567,753	69	40	49	39
Malta	5,696					5,391	77	63	80	86	4,696		94	74	94
Mauritania	67,195					88,396	79	33	38	33	116,539	75	40	62	44
Mauritius	23,630	89	89		90	21,506	87	85	76	86	18,758	88	88	84	88

* Measles containing vaccine (M, MR, MMR)
** 3 doses of polio vaccine (OPV or IPV)

Country	1980 Births	BCG	DTP3	*MCV	**Pol3	1990 Births	BCG	DTP3	*MCV	**Pol3	2000 Births	BCG	DTP3	*MCV	**Pol3
Mexico	2,309,597	48	44	35	91	2,345,712	70	66	78	96	2,309,792	99	97	97	89
Mongolia	63,845	51	76	17	86	71,630	81	84	92	87	57,564	97	95	94	94
Morocco	742,961					757,800	96	81	80	81	772,982	99	95	93	95
Mozambique	544,633					635,110	59	46	59	46	793,043	99	88	97	87
Myanmar	1,219,256	9	4			1,249,097	95	88	90	88	1,185,704	88	82	84	86
Namibia	41,666					57,358	85	53	41	54	62,956	77	79	69	80
Nepal	573,853	22	8			697,212	74	43	57	42	812,125	84	72	71	92
Netherlands	171,903		96	91	96	193,411		97	94	97	178,777		97	96	97
New Zealand	50,785		76	80		58,628		90	90	90	53,666		90	85	82
Nicaragua	135,386	33	15	15	21	147,371	84	66	82	87	171,863	96	93	99	93
Niger	319,883					428,710	50	22	25	22	603,723	54	31	34	31
Nigeria	3,069,867					3,872,051	80	56	54	55	4,627,568	54	26	40	25
Norway	50,115					58,755	94	86	87	84	54,816	98	95	92	96
Oman	51,224	51	18	22	18	74,387	96	98	98	98	90,114	98	99	99	99
Pakistan	3,502,446	6	2	1	2	4,464,300	80	54	50	54	5,241,841	78	56	54	58
Panama	57,474	68	47	71	44	62,846	97	86	73	86	60,996	99	98	97	99
Papua New Guinea	117,507	62	32		29	142,916	89	67	67	67	157,995	70	57	68	46
Paraguay	115,967	31	17	17	13	149,198	75	67	69	64	167,221	51	66	77	63
Peru	621,926	57	16	23	16	626,780	83	72	64	73	607,648	93	91	97	89
Philippines	1,757,772	56	47		50	2,004,560	96	88	85	88	2,058,729	81	79	80	75
Poland	702,631	93	96	92	96	554,382	97	96	95	96	375,803	96	98	97	98
Portugal	162,001		73	54	18	115,949	88	89	85	89	112,664	82	96	87	96
Qatar	7,150	4	61	26	61	10,045	97	82	79	82	10,589	99	90	87	90
Republic of Korea	850,096			4		693,301	72	74	93	74	612,739	73	97	95	99
Republic of Moldova	0	92	88	94	94	0	96	81	94	91	50,166	98	91	87	92
Romania	384,472					319,787	90	96	92	92	231,994	99	99	98	99
Russian Federation	0					0					1,235,727	96	95	97	97
Rwanda	268,590					265,162	92	84	83	83	301,746	81	90	74	90
Saint Lucia	3,670	27	56		58	3,349	97	91	83	90	3,460	91	70	95	70
Sao Tome and Principe	0					0	99	92	71	90	0	81	82	69	87
Saudi Arabia	415,651	33	41	8	50	588,603	90	92	88	92	694,502	94	95	94	95
Senegal	268,215					318,020	90	51	51	53	363,780	89	52	48	49
Seychelles	0					0	98	99	86	99	0	99	98	97	98
Sierra Leone	157,875					195,789					224,477	74	44	37	46
Singapore	40,415	85	84	47	83	54,162	99	85	84	85	49,334	98	93	91	93
Slovakia	0					0					55,522	94	99	98	98

* Measles containing vaccine (M, MR, MMR)

** 3 doses of polio vaccine (OPV or IPV)

Country	1980 Births	BCG	DTP3	*MCV	**Pol3	1990 Births	BCG	DTP3	*MCV	**Pol3	2000 Births	BCG	DTP3	*MCV	**Pol3
Slovenia	0		89	85	87	0		95	84	95	17,201	96	92	98	93
Somalia	312,679	6		9	8	364,796	31	19	30	18	461,168	69	33	38	37
South Africa	1,008,691					1,032,428	57	72	79	76	1,113,771	99	79	77	76
Spain	576,266					405,143		93	97	94	359,625		95	94	95
Sri Lanka	400,758	61	46		46	355,843	84	86	80	86	325,893	99	99	99	99
Sudan	826,460	2	1		1	958,940	77	62	57	62	1,089,529	46	41	47	41
Suriname	10,857		25	1	24	9,462		83	65	81	8,058		85	85	84
Swaziland	24,218					30,186	96	89	85	89	31,633	90	77	72	76
Sweden	92,853					117,822		99	95	99	77,679		99	96	99
Switzerland	71,818					81,889		90	90	98	67,221		189	162	190
Syrian Arab Republic	403,542	35	13	13	13	466,628	92	90	87	90	484,422	99	94	94	94
Tajikistan	0					0					155,476	99	83	87	85
TFYRM	0					0					26,492	97	95	97	96
Thailand	1,288,543	68	49		19	1,133,569	99	92	80	92	1,182,072	99	97	94	97
Togo	118,399					147,967	97	77	73	76	178,114	84	64	58	63
Trinidad and Tobago	32,029		26		38	24,944		89	99	89	17,353		90	90	90
Tunisia	230,931					229,602	96	93	93	93	171,165	97	96	85	96
Turkey	1,497,768		42	27	63	1,594,344	93	84	78	84	1,451,523	89	85	86	85
Turkmenistan	0					0					127,077	99	97	97	98
Uganda	629,177					870,897	75	45	52	45	1,183,622	77	53	56	53
Ukraine	0					0					409,952	99	99	99	99
United Arab Emirates	30,536	15	11	34	11	46,723	96	85	80	85	40,513	98	94	94	94
United Kingdom	699,670		41	53	81	780,283		84	87	92	667,824		94	87	95
United Republic of Tanzania	883,309	72	59	46	57	1,146,002	85	78	80	78	1,379,016	86	79	78	64
United States of America	3,532,862		96	86	95	4,060,757		90	90	85	3,880,477		94	91	90
Uruguay	55,928	56	53	50	59	56,789	99	97	97	97	57,651	99	90	89	92
USSR	4,983,039					4,854,399	90	68	85	74	0				
Uzbekistan	0					0	94	87	85	90	545,100	98	96	99	96
Vanuatu	4,667					5,541					6,394	99	90	94	87
Venezuela	498,244		56	50	95	563,277	74	61	61	71	575,281	99	86	84	86
Viet Nam	1,850,966					2,041,524	90	85	85	85	1,575,632	94	96	97	96
Yemen	424,239	9	1	2	1	603,870	95	84	69	84	925,918	82	76	71	76
Yugoslavia	378,526					319,674	97	84	83	81	123,427	99	95	89	98
Zambia	271,729					361,190	97	91	90	90	443,755	92	78	85	79
Zimbabwe	321,391					424,540	91	88	87	89	455,787	82	77	70	70

* Measles containing vaccine (M, MR, MMR)

** 3 doses of polio vaccine (OPV or IPV)

DTP3 coverage, 2001

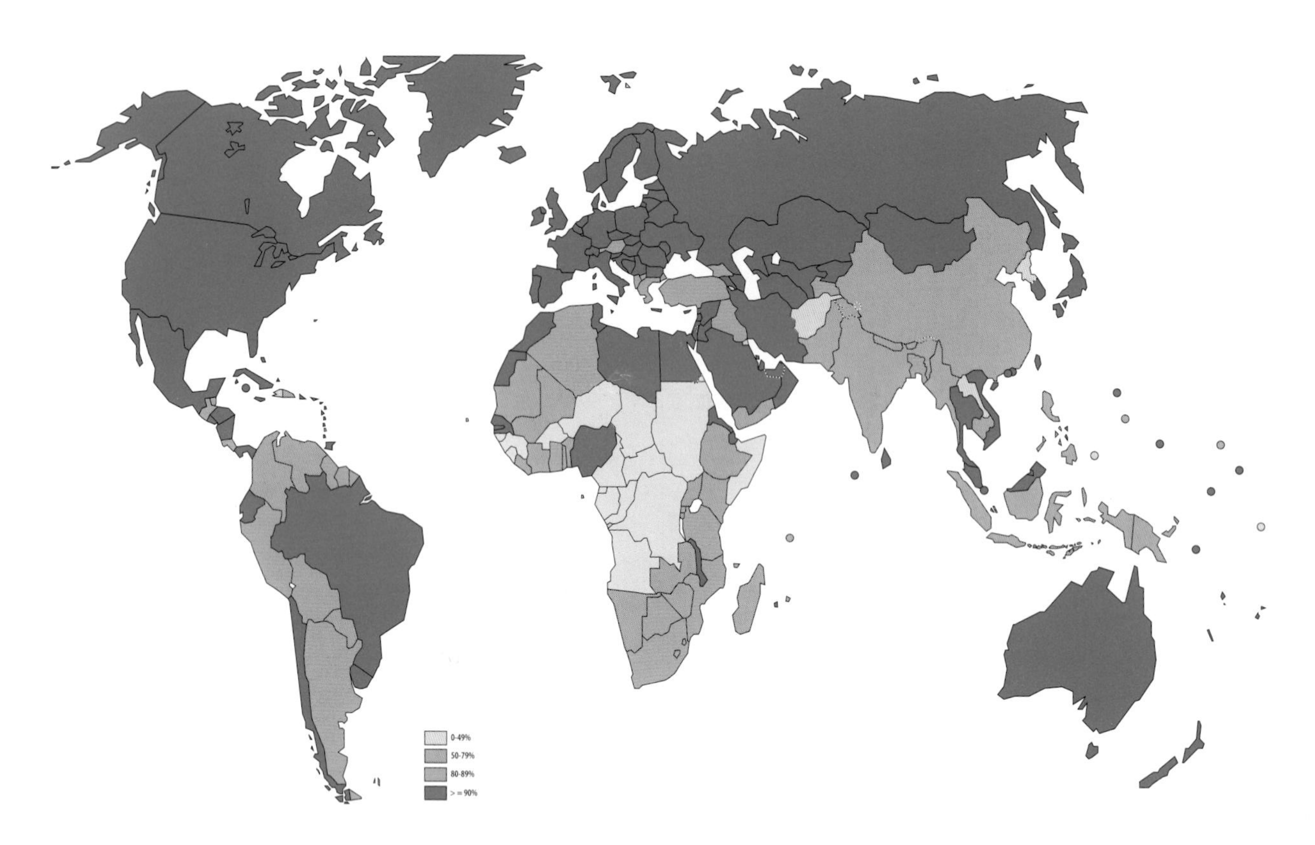

The boundaries and names shown and the designations used on this map do not imply the expression of any opinion whatsoever on the part of the World health Organization concerning the legal status of any country, territory, city or area or of its authorities, or concerning the delimitation of its frontiers or boundaries. Dotted lines on maps represent approximate border lines for which there may not yet be full agreement.

Source: WHO/UNICEF estimates 2002

Of the five major meningococcal serogroups – A, B, C, W135, and Y – the first three are responsible for most cases worldwide. Serogroup A meningococcal disease occurs in explosive epidemics along the sub-Saharan "meningitis belt" in irregular cycles every 5–12 years, with over 200 million people in 18 countries at risk. The highest disease rates occur among young children, but in epidemics, teenagers and young adults are also affected. Serogroups B and C are most common in the developed world during endemic periods. These cause occasional epidemics but not on the scale of those caused by serogroup A meningococcus.

In 1996, in one of the largest outbreaks of serogroup A meningococcal meningitis ever recorded in Africa, there were at least 200 000 cases and 20 000 deaths. The epidemic stretched vaccine supplies to their limit. This led to the establishment in 1997 of the WHO-brokered International Coordinating Group (ICG), an inter-agency mechanism which monitors the incidence of meningitis and coordinates the emergency supply and fair distribution of meningitis vaccine to protect the populations most at risk. This group estimates vaccine needs and oversees the purchase and distribution of high quality vaccine and safe injection equipment. Countries are offered vaccine from an emergency stockpile at a preferential price.

More recently in Africa, there has been an alarming upsurge in cases involving the W135 strains, previously endemic but now emerging in epidemic form. As of early May 2002, an epidemic in Burkina Faso involved over 12 000 cases and more than 1400 deaths. The outbreak spread to 17 districts, putting 7 million people at risk. Authorities were unprepared for an outbreak of this size and global stocks of the W135-containing tetravalent polysaccharide vaccine were inadequate to protect the population at risk. Only two manufacturers, Aventis Pasteur and GlaxoSmithKline, currently produce the tetravalent vaccine and, unless current production capacity can be increased, adequate supplies will not be available for two to three years. An additional problem is that the vaccine is too expensive for most low-income countries. On behalf of the ICG, WHO has engaged with vaccine manufacturers and public health officials to mitigate the current vaccine crisis and to establish a future stockpile of the tetravalent vaccine to meet long-term needs.

Vaccine update

Polysaccharide vaccines are available to protect against serogroups A and C (bivalent), or against serogroups A, C, W135, and Y (tetravalent). Although these vaccines provide only short-term immunity and have variable effectiveness among children under two years, they are essential during epidemics to protect the populations at risk. A new vaccine is urgently needed to prevent epidemics of the disease in sub-Saharan Africa. The ideal vaccine would provide longer-term protection at all ages and reduce transmission of meningococcus in the population, thereby establishing what is known as "herd immunity". Experience with both Hib and pneumococcal conjugate vaccines and, more recently, with serogroup C meningococcal conjugate vaccines in the UK, indicates that a conjugate vaccine targeted for prevention of serogroup A meningococcal disease could prevent most epidemic meningococcal disease in Africa.

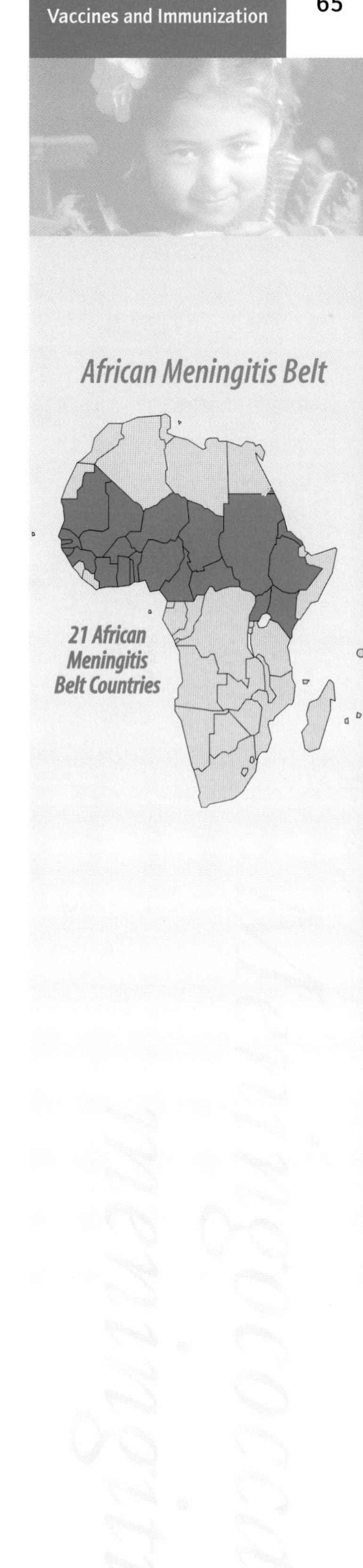

A prototype serogroup A and C meningococcal conjugate vaccine has already been tested in African children and was found to be safe and effective, and capable of priming for long-term immunity. However, due to the lack of a guaranteed market for this product, by 1999 all vaccine manufacturers had halted their development programmes for serogroup A/C conjugate vaccines and moved to developing alternative combinations instead.

Meanwhile, efforts to develop a vaccine against serogroup B meningococcus, which accounts for the majority of cases in Europe and the United States, have been unsuccessful. Protein vaccines have been 50–80% effective and were successful in controlling epidemics in Brazil, Cuba and Norway, but they fail to protect the very young, and immunity also wanes over time. Elsewhere, trials in Chile and Iceland have shown these vaccines to be most effective against single rather than multiple strains. However, following the successful sequencing of the meningococcal genome, the recent discovery of several new proteins has raised the potential for new candidate vaccines.

Since the incidence of rotavirus disease is similar among children in developing and developed countries, it is unlikely that improvements in hygiene and sanitation will suffice to prevent the disease

Rotavirus diarrhoea

Disease burden

Rotavirus is the leading cause of severe, dehydrating diarrhoea in children worldwide. It accounts for about one-third of all hospital admissions for diarrhoeal disease, and 500 000–600 000 deaths a year among children under five, mainly in developing countries. Most children throughout the world have been infected by the age of five.

In the United States, the economic costs of rotavirus disease are estimated at US$ 1 billion a year, including US$ 300 million in health care costs. Since the incidence of rotavirus disease is similar among children in developing and developed countries, it is unlikely that improvements in hygiene and sanitation will suffice to prevent the disease. While rotavirus diarrhoea can be considerably reduced with appropriate rehydration therapy, the best strategy would be to prevent rotavirus infection by vaccination.

Vaccine update

Several approaches have been used to develop rotavirus vaccines. The leading candidate vaccines are live, oral preparations based on either attenuated human rotaviruses or on genetically engineered vaccines combining elements of human and animal rotaviruses.

In 1998, a genetically engineered vaccine, rhesus rotavirus vaccine-tetravalent (RRV-TV), was developed by Wyeth-Lederle and licensed in the United States. However, the vaccine was withdrawn within a year of licensure because it was associated with intussusception (a telescoping bowel condition) in approximately one in 10 000–12 000 infants vaccinated. Wyeth-Lederle stopped production of the vaccine in 1999, leaving a void in the introduction of the vaccine in Europe, Latin America and the developing world.

Several candidate rotavirus vaccines are currently in development and are being tested. GlaxoSmithKline is developing a vaccine based on an attenuated human rotavirus. Initial Phase 1 and II trials showed the vaccine to be effective, and the vaccine is currently being tested (including Phase III efficacy trials) in different regions of the world. Merck is developing a rotavirus vaccine that includes genes for the most common serotypes of rotavirus globally. This vaccine is currently being tested for safety and efficacy in large-scale clinical trials in Finland and the United States.

Several local manufacturers are also developing rotavirus vaccines. In China, a vaccine based on a lamb rotavirus strain is currently licensed and being used. In India, vaccines based on two naturally occurring strains of rotavirus are being developed, and a vaccine based on a neonatal human strain of rotavirus from Australia is also being developed. Other approaches to vaccines, including inactivated rotavirus vaccines and DNA vaccines, are being pursued but are in relatively early stages of development.

With support from the Children's Vaccine Program at PATH, GAVI is accelerating the development of rotavirus vaccines as a priority for developing countries. Because of the experience with RRV-TV, WHO has recommended that multinational companies developing rotavirus vaccines test these simultaneously in both developing and developed countries, and that future trials should include active surveillance for intussusception.

4. Neglected vaccines

- **Shigella dysentery**
- **Dengue**
- **Japanese encephalitis**
- **Leishmaniasis**
- **Schistosomiasis**
- **Cholera**

A number of diseases which occur mainly in developing countries and account for a high disease burden, currently offer poor financial incentives to major pharmaceutical manufacturers. These include diseases such as schistosomiasis and leishmaniasis. With only a limited potential market for these vaccines among the developed countries, e.g. travellers and military personnel, there is little leeway for offsetting lower prices in developing countries against the higher prices obtainable in the wealthier countries. Without support from the public sector and commitments to purchase new vaccines once available, R&D of these vaccines will not be accelerated. In the meantime, an increase in drug resistance and coinfection with HIV are today undermining efforts to treat some of these diseases.

Without support from the public sector and commitments to purchase new vaccines once available, R&D of these vaccines will not be accelerated

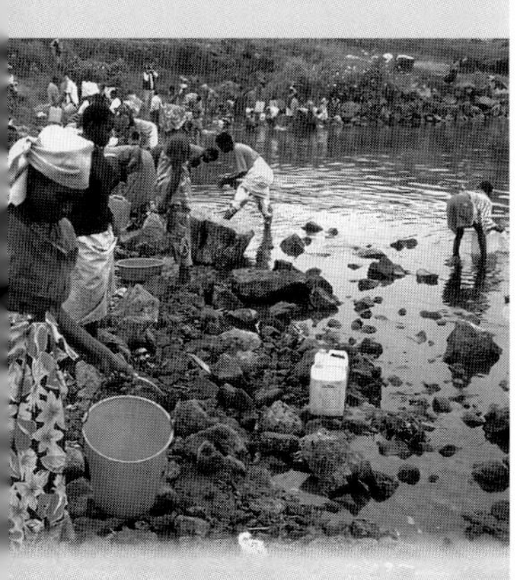

The disease thrives in conditions of poverty, especially where there is overcrowding, poor sanitation and no access to safe water

Shigella dysentery

Disease burden

Shigella dysentery is a major cause of death among young children in the developing world. In countries where the disease is endemic, it accounts for 10% of all cases of diarrhoeal disease among children under five.

The disease is highly contagious and can occur in explosive epidemics with major loss of life. It thrives in conditions of poverty, especially where there is overcrowding, poor sanitation and no access to safe water. The disease also occurs in developed countries, especially where hygiene is poor.

Although the disease can be treated with antibiotics and oral rehydration therapy, the disease-causing shigellae are increasingly resistant to antibiotics and multidrug-resistant strains (both endemic and epidemic) are now widespread.

Since the 1960s, pandemics have occurred in Central America, South and South-East Asia, and sub-Saharan Africa. The disease often strikes populations during times of political upheaval and natural disaster, due to the consequent decline of living conditions. For several months in 1994, shigella dysentery was the main cause of death in Rwandan refugee camps in Burundi, Tanzania and Zaire. Over a single month in Zaire, 20 000 refugees died after contracting shigella caused by a strain of the bacterium that was resistant to all the commonly-used antibiotics. Shigella dysentery is also an increasing problem among populations infected with HIV. Coinfection with the two diseases leads to a more severe form of shigella dysentery, including persistent or recurrent intestinal disease and bacteraemia.

The disease burden can be reduced by improvements to water supplies and sanitation, while drug resistance can be slowed by a more rational prescribing of antibiotics. A vaccine that could protect against both sensitive and drug-resistant strains of the bacterium would have the biggest impact on efforts to control the disease.

Vaccine update

Biotechnological advances have led to a new generation of candidate vaccines, some of which are dependent on antibiotics, and others derived from wild type *Shigella*. It is a complicated bacterium with many subtypes. The main strain in the developing and the developed world is *S. flexneri* subtype 2a. The challenge is to incorporate relevant strains so that the vaccine prevents the most dangerous and explosive strains in addition to those most resistant to drugs. There are four different bacterial groups which divide into 47 different serotypes, some of which are rare and account for very few cases; some are more resistant to drugs than others; and others account for the majority of cases in developing countries but are rarely found in the developed world.

The ideal vaccine would be a polyvalent cocktail vaccine which includes *S. sonnei,* responsible for 15% of infections in developing countries and 77% in developed countries; *S. dysenteriae,* which, although rare, can cause pandemics, is

Shigella dysentery

multidrug-resistant, causes high attack rates and is often fatal; and *S. flexneri* which accounts for 60% of cases in developing countries.

With six major serotypes, *S. flexneri* poses a unique challenge to the vaccine formulation. A vaccine covering all *S. flexneri* serotypes, *S. sonnei* and *S. dysenteriae* serotype 1 (the epidemic serotype) could be expected to protect against an estimated 79% of shigella infections in developing countries and 83% in developed countries, preventing 91million infections (over 90 million in developing countries and almost 1 million in developed countries) and 605 000 deaths each year. Of candidate vaccines in development, injectable conjugate vaccines against *S. flexneri* 2a and *S. sonnei* plus a live attenuated *S. flexneri* 2a oral vaccine candidate are the most advanced. These vaccines have undergone limited testing in Bangladesh and Israel, but further trials are still required. It is likely to be 5–10 years before a vaccine is introduced. The main participants in shigella vaccine development are the Pasteur Institute, Paris; U.S. National Institutes of Health, Washington D.C.; Center for Vaccine Development, University of Maryland School of Medicine, Baltimore; Walter Reed Army Institute of Research, Washington; International Vaccine Institute, Seoul; and WHO.

Dengue

Disease burden

Dengue is a mosquito-borne viral infection that has spread alarmingly over the past three decades. WHO estimates that there may be 50 million cases of dengue infection worldwide every year. Between 1970 and 1995, the number of countries to experience epidemics of the more serious dengue haemorrhagic fever increased four-fold to include more than 100 countries in Africa, the Americas, the Eastern Mediterranean, South-East Asia and the Western Pacific. About 2.5 billion people are believed to be potentially at risk.

Aedes aegypti; **adult female mosquito taking a blood meal on human skin**

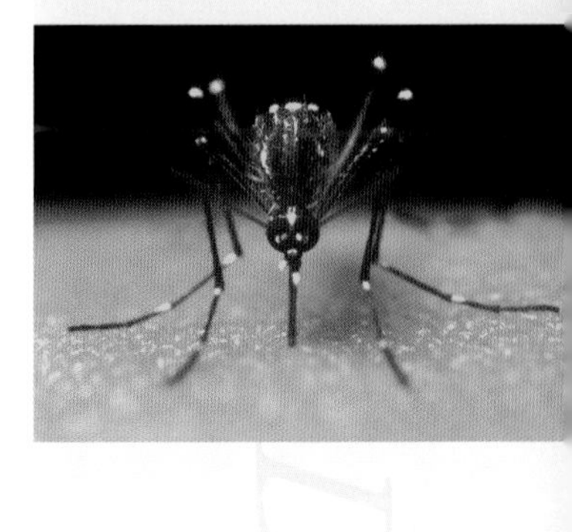

The increase in cases is the result of the expanding geographical distribution of the mosquitos which carry the virus, especially the *Aedes aegypti* species which is mainly found in urban areas. At the same time, the rapid rise in urban populations has increased the number of people exposed to the virus.

Dengue is a flu-like illness that rarely causes death. It is caused by one of four dengue viruses. Recovery from infection ensures lifelong immunity against the particular virus involved, but not against the other three. Even worse, if subsequent infection with a different serotype occurs, it is believed to increase susceptibility to dengue haemorrhagic fever – a life-threatening condition which particularly affects young children and has a 20% fatality rate if left untreated. An estimated 500 000 cases of dengue haemorrhagic fever require hospitalization every year. This form of the disease is also on the increase.

Although there is no specific cure for dengue fever, intensive hospital-based nursing care, including fluid replacement, can prevent most deaths. In the absence of a vaccine, environmental management (to reduce the number of mosquito breeding places) and vector control are at present the only means of preventing and controlling the disease.

Dengue

Vaccine update

Many biotechnological approaches have been used in attempts to develop dengue vaccine candidates, including live attenuated vaccines, infectious clone-derived vaccines, recombinant live vector systems, subunit vaccines and nucleic acid vaccines. Further trials, licensing and introduction could take between seven and 10 years before a vaccine becomes available.

The current candidates are two tetravalent live attenuated vaccines developed in Thailand and the United States, both of which are now in clinical trials. The Thai vaccine was originally developed at Mahidol University, Bangkok, with the support of WHO, and then provided to Pasteur Merieux Connaught (now Aventis Pasteur) for production on an industrial scale. A Phase II clinical trial is now in progress in Thailand. The second dengue tetravalent live attenuated vaccine candidate was developed at the Walter Reed Army Institute for Research, United States, where a Phase II clinical trial is being prepared. Chimeric vaccines are also in development, combining infectious clones of dengue and a vaccine strain of yellow fever. This work was initiated by St Louis University, United States, with grant support from WHO, and moved into development by Oravax/Acambis, in the United States. Other manufacturers and researchers include the Hawaii Biotechnology Group, CDC, and NIH.

An estimated 2.4 billion people in parts of Asia and the Pacific region are at risk of Japanese encephalitis

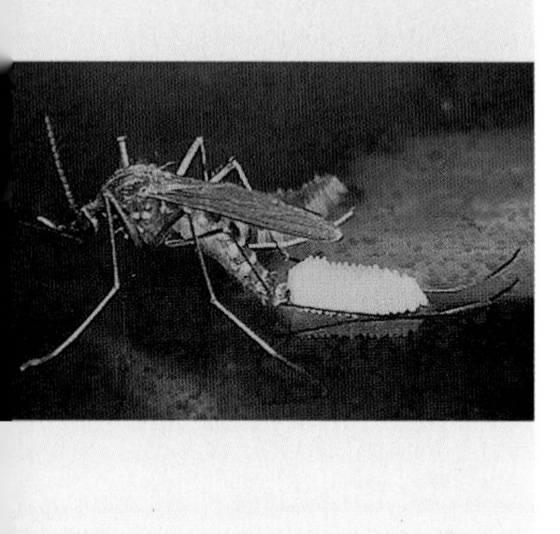

Japanese encephalitis

Disease burden

An estimated 2.4 billion people in parts of Asia and the Pacific region are at risk of Japanese encephalitis, a mosquito-borne viral disease with a high fatality rate. There are over 50 000 reported cases of the disease every year and approximately 4000 deaths. Up to one-third of survivors suffer severe neurological damage including paralysis and brain damage. Most deaths and long-term disability occur among children under 10. If the disease is contracted during the early stages of pregnancy there is a high risk of miscarriage.

The disease occurs mainly in rural agricultural areas, where pools of water or flooded rice fields provide a breeding ground for mosquitos. The mosquito transmits the virus to humans after biting an infected animal. Pigs, wading birds and ducks are all potential carriers of the virus. In recent decades, outbreaks of Japanese encephalitis have occurred in previously non-endemic areas. There have also been outbreaks among urban populations in several major Asian cities. In the worst-affected areas, Japanese encephalitis is a significant public health burden with high social and economic costs. No effective antiviral drugs are available to treat the disease.

Japanese encephalitis

Vaccine update

More than forty years ago, an inactivated vaccine against Japanese encephalitis was developed in Japan. The vaccine has dramatically reduced the incidence of Japanese encephalitis in the Democratic People's Republic of Korea, Japan, Republic of Korea and Taiwan, China. However, production capacity is limited, the vaccine offers only short-term protection and there have been reports of neurological reactions (all in European settings) after vaccination.

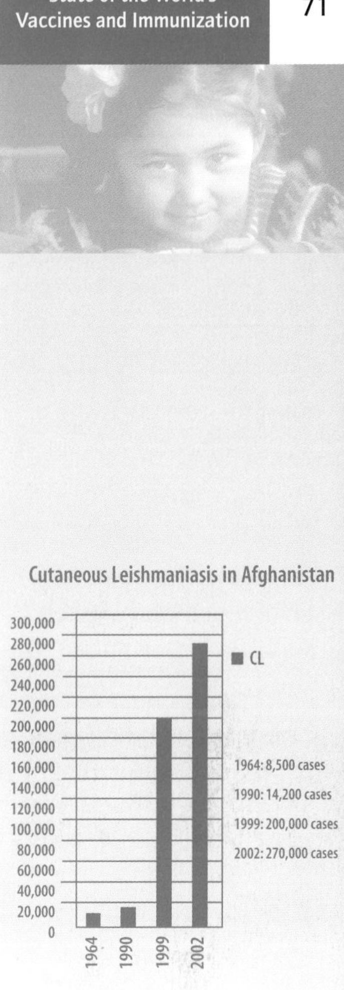

A live attenuated vaccine has been developed and tested in China. This appears to be safe and effective in immunization programmes involving millions of children and has successfully controlled the disease there, but it is not yet suitable for global use. Novel inactivated vaccines derived from virus grown in tissue culture are also being developed and have shown encouraging results in Phase I clinical trials.

A chimeric yellow fever/Japanese encephalitis vaccine candidate has also shown promising results in Phase I clinical trials. This candidate vaccine involves the use of the yellow fever vaccine as a vector to deliver antigenic Japanese encephalitis proteins. These vectors induce both cellular and antibody immunity against the virus and could hold promise for the future. With further clinical testing and licensing it will be at least five years before this vaccine is commercially introduced. The main manufacturers and researchers on Japanese encephalitis vaccines are Acambis (UK and United States), Biken (Japan), Chemo-Sero Therapeutic Research Institute (Japan), the National Institutes of Health (United States), the National Vaccine and Serum Institute (China), CDC and the Walter Reed Army Institute of Research (United States).

Leishmaniasis

Disease burden

Leishmaniasis – a devastating parasitic disease with the capacity to maim and kill – is on the increase worldwide. Since 1993, the geographical spread of the disease has increased and there has been a sharp rise in the number of recorded cases. Over 12 million people are infected and there are an estimated 1.5–2 million cases of the disease every year. In 2000, there were 41 000 deaths due to leishmaniasis. There have been recent epidemics of the disease in a number of countries, including India and Sudan, and about 350 million people are currently at risk in 88 countries in Africa, Asia, Europe, and North and South America.

The upsurge in cases has been fuelled by an increase in the spread of the sandfly vector (mainly due to changes in land and water use, including deforestation and dam construction), population movements to and from endemic areas, and by the soaring rates of HIV infection, which increases susceptibility to visceral leishmaniasis, a life-threatening form of the disease.

Of the 1–1.5 million annual cases of cutaneous leishmaniasis (the most common form of the disease, which ulcerates the face, arms and legs) 90% occur in Afghanistan, Brazil, Peru and Syria. Of the 500 000 annual cases of visceral leishmaniasis, 90% occur in Bangladesh, India, Nepal and Sudan. The mucocutaneous form of the disease (which disfigures the nose, mouth and throat) occurs mainly in Bolivia, Brazil and Peru.

In areas where visceral leishmaniasis is endemic, coinfection with HIV has led to the emergence of a new life-threatening condition. People infected with HIV have a dramatically increased risk – at least 100-fold – of developing visceral leishmaniasis when exposed to the parasite. In turn, visceral leishmaniasis accelerates the onset of AIDS, triggering opportunistic infections such as TB and pneumonia, and shortening life expectancy. The disease can also be transmitted person-to-person by sharing injecting equipment, which accounts for an upsurge in the disease in south-western Europe (Spain, Italy, France and Portugal) among injecting drug-users.

Although visceral leishmaniasis can be treated, the parasite is increasingly resistant to first-line treatment which involves several weeks of injections with pentavalent antimonial drugs. In India, which accounts for about half of all cases worldwide, 40% of cases are now resistant. While second-line drugs exist, they involve lengthy infusions over four to six weeks in special treatment centres. The medication is toxic and most patients suffer unpleasant, occasionally life-threatening, side-effects. The very high cost of treatment also puts the medication way beyond the reach of the people most affected, most of them poor.

Phlebotomus dubasci a sandfly vector of leishmania parasites, taking a blood meal through human skin

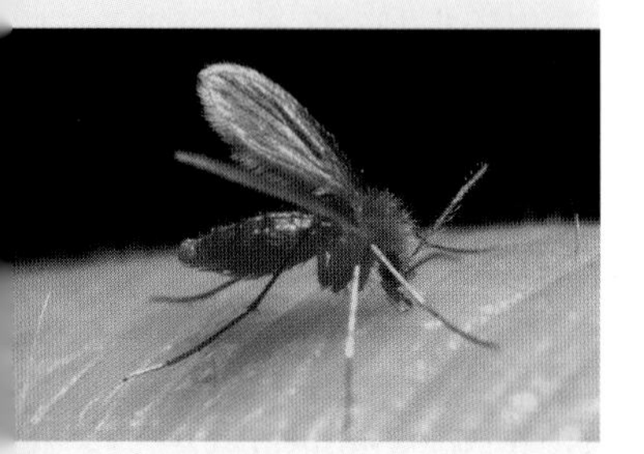

A new oral treatment (miltefosine) has been successfully tested among adults in India and has now been licensed for use there through a public-private partnership involving the UNDP/World Bank/WHO Special Programme for Research and Training in Tropical Diseases (TDR) and a private manufacturer (Zentaris). Trials of the drug among children are still under way. In the longer-term, a vaccine offers the best hope of controlling the different forms of the disease.

Vaccine update

Leishmaniasis vaccine development remains fragmented and lacks the backing of a large international pharmaceutical industry partner capable of bringing the product to market. Nevertheless, there is hope that a vaccine can be developed to protect against both cutaneous and visceral leishmaniasis.

A number of first-generation candidates have entered human trials and have been shown to be partially effective. In the Islamic Republic of Iran, for example, a potential vaccine against cutaneous leishmaniasis succeeded in boosting immunity (more effectively in boys than girls), although it did not confer significant protection. WHO is currently supporting further clinical trials in Colombia, in the Islamic Republic of Iran (in partnership with Teheran University), and in Sudan with the Institute for Endemic Diseases, Khartoum. Elsewhere, a cutaneous leishmaniasis therapeutic vaccine has also recently been registered in Brazil.

WHO and the Infectious Disease Research Institute (IDRI) of Washington State University, United States, have played a major role in research efforts to date. A donation of US$ 15 million from the Bill & Melinda Gates Foundation to IDRI is supporting the R&D of second generation vaccines, one of which has recently entered Phase I trials. Despite this progress, an effective vaccine is still about 5–12 years away.

Schistosomiasis

Disease burden

Schistosomiasis is the second most prevalent tropical disease after malaria, afflicting an estimated 200 million people in over 70 countries. Most cases (85%) occur in Africa, but schistosomiasis also poses a serious health threat in parts of Latin America and Asia. The disease accounts for 11 000 deaths a year worldwide, and an estimated 600 million people are at risk worldwide.

The disease is contracted through contact with the disease-causing schistosomes – snail-borne parasites – in stagnant water. Young children are often the worst affected. Without treatment – an annual dose of the drug praziquantel – schistosomiasis can lead to chronic urinary tract infection, cirrhosis of the liver and bladder cancer.

Schistosomiasis is an increasing public health problem in areas where changes in land use such as deforestation, agricultural development, dams and irrigation schemes have led to the proliferation of the snails that harbour the parasites. In the worst-affected areas, the disease exerts a heavy social and economic toll on populations. The onset of schistosomiasis-related anaemia and chronic fatigue account for a high percentage of missed schooling and lost working days.

Efforts to control the disease include the destruction of snails and snail habitats, and annual population-wide treatment with praziquantel. However environmental control has been only partially successful, drug treatment is not 100% effective and there are already reports of drug-resistance in some areas. A safe and cost-effective vaccine is the optimal way to control the disease in the long term.

Vaccine update

Schistosomiasis continues to outwit the scientific community and has so far failed to attract significant interest from any of the major vaccine manufacturers. Two leading candidate vaccines been successful in animal models. One of these, a protein recombinant vaccine candidate (the Sh-GST molecule) is in advanced Phase II large-scale human trials in Niger and Senegal. Developed at the Pasteur Institute in France, it is designed to protect against both the *Schistosoma haematobium* strain (most common in Africa) and the *S. mansoni* strain (found in Africa and South America). The other vaccine candidate, based on paramyosin (an invertebrate muscle protein worked on at NIH), is expected to enter clinical trials in the near future. Several candidates against *S. japonicum* (a strain found mainly in China and the Philippines) are also nearing clinical testing. Major funding agencies for these projects are the European Union and WHO/TDR.

The Schistosomiasis Vaccine Development Project (SVDP) is supported by USAID in Egypt and is a direct follow-up to previous separate research projects on an *S. mansoni* vaccine supported by USAID, WHO and NIH. These developments resulted in a shortlist of six priority molecules recommended for further research. There are currently two antigens ready for scaling up: paramyosin (from NIH) and Sm-14 (a fatty acid binding protein developed at FIOCRUZ in Brazil). An effective vaccine is about 7–12 years away.

Water contact point: a young woman uses a backpack spray to water the vegetables she is growing in her fields. She exposes herself to infection when she fills up the backpack sprayer with water from the nearby pond

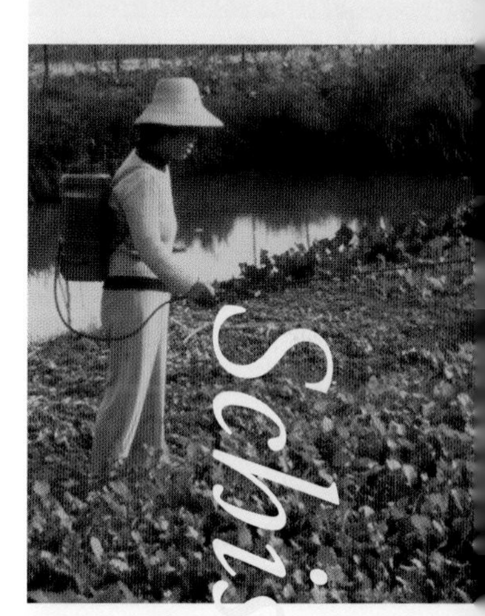

Cholera

Disease burden

Every year an estimated 120 000 people die from cholera due to severe dehydration and vomiting. In 2001, the number of reported cases (only a fraction of the estimated number) increased by one-third, with 94% of cases reported in Africa.

Cholera occurs, often in explosive epidemics, in areas where sanitation is inadequate, access to safe drinking water is limited, and personal hygiene is poor. Caused by a bacterium *(Vibrio cholerae)* and contracted mainly through consumption of contaminated food or drinking water, the disease disproportionately affects the poor in developing countries throughout the world. Among the most vulnerable populations are the victims of complex emergencies – including refugees and displaced persons – and people living in overcrowded slums or makeshift dwellings in shanty towns. In 1994, in the aftermath of the conflict in Rwanda, an outbreak of cholera in the overcrowded refugee camps in Goma, former Zaire, killed almost 24 000 people in a single month.

The ongoing cholera pandemic – the seventh since records began in the early 19th century – originated in Indonesia in 1961 and has since spread to over 100 countries throughout the world. The current pandemic is caused by *V. cholerae* 01 (the so-called El Tor biotype) which is responsible for the majority of cholera cases worldwide. A new serogroup, 0139, was discovered in Bangladesh in 1992, but it is not yet known whether this strain could also cause a pandemic.

In countries with poorly developed disease surveillance and reporting systems, cholera cases often go undetected until a major outbreak occurs. To make matters worse, many countries are reluctant to report cholera cases for fear of attracting unwarranted international trade restrictions or the loss of tourist revenues. A 1991 outbreak of the disease in Peru is estimated to have cost US$ 770 million in lost revenues, mainly due to food embargoes and lost tourism. Elsewhere in the United Republic of Tanzania estimated losses of US$ 36 million were incurred during an outbreak in 1998.

The disease can be prevented through the improvement of personal hygiene (especially hand-washing), by ensuring that food is safely prepared and that water is made safe by boiling or treatment, and in the longer-term, by the improvement of sanitation and the provision of safe drinking water. In addition, a low-cost intervention, oral rehydration, exists to treat those affected. With rapid and effective treatment less than 1% of cholera patients die. However, where treatment is not available, as many as 50% of those affected may die.

Vaccine update

Three cholera vaccines, which have been shown to be safe and effective, are currently available. These vaccines have been licensed in some countries and are used mainly by travellers. However, oral cholera vaccines are now under consideration for public health use in emergency situations to immunize populations considered at high risk of a cholera outbreak.

One vaccine consists of killed whole cell *V. cholerae* 01 with purified recombinant B-subunit of cholera toxoid (WC/rB). Field trials in Bangladesh, Peru and Sweden have shown that this vaccine is safe, immunogenic and effective, and confers 85–90% protection for six months in all age groups after administration of two doses, one or two weeks apart. This vaccine is licenced in Norway, Sweden, the United States and in some Latin American countries.

As a result of technology transfer, a variant of the WC/rB vaccine containing no recombinant B-subunit has been produced and tested in Viet Nam. It is administered in two doses, one week apart. A field trial conducted in 1992–1993 in Viet Nam, showed an efficacy of 66% against El Tor at 8 months in all age groups. The vaccine is licensed only in Viet Nam but is also being produced in Indonesia.

Another oral vaccine consists of a live attenuated genetically modified *V. cholerae* 01 strain (CVD 103-HgR), produced in Switzerland. Placebo-controlled trials in a number of countries in Asia and South America have shown the safety and immunogenicity of a single dose of this vaccine. It is licensed in Australia, Canada, New Zealand, Switzerland and several Latin American countries.

Another live attenuated vaccine developed in Cuba (one oral dose) has been tested in Phase 1 trials.

4. Other vaccines

- **Cervical cancer (human papillomavirus)**
- **Respiratory syncytial virus (RSV)**
- **Herpes simplex virus type 2**
- ***Enterotoxigenic Escherichia coli* (ETEC)**

While *State of the World's Vaccines and Immunization* does not include comprehensive coverage of all new vaccines currently in the vaccine research and development pipeline, it includes a range of vaccines of key public health importance. This section looks at progress in the discovery of new vaccines to prevent four additional high-burden diseases.

Cervical cancer (human papillomavirus)

Disease burden

Worldwide, cervical cancer is the third most common cancer among women after breast cancer and cancer of the colon/rectum.* Most cases are caused by infection with different types of human papillomavirus (HPV), a highly contagious virus which is also associated with common skin warts, genital warts and anogenital cancer.

It is estimated that approximately 630 million people are infected with HPV, the most commonly diagnosed viral cause of sexually transmitted infections.

** Cervical cancer is the 2nd most common cancer among women in developing countries and the 6th most common in developed countries.*

There are an estimated 510 000 new cases of cervical cancer worldwide every year

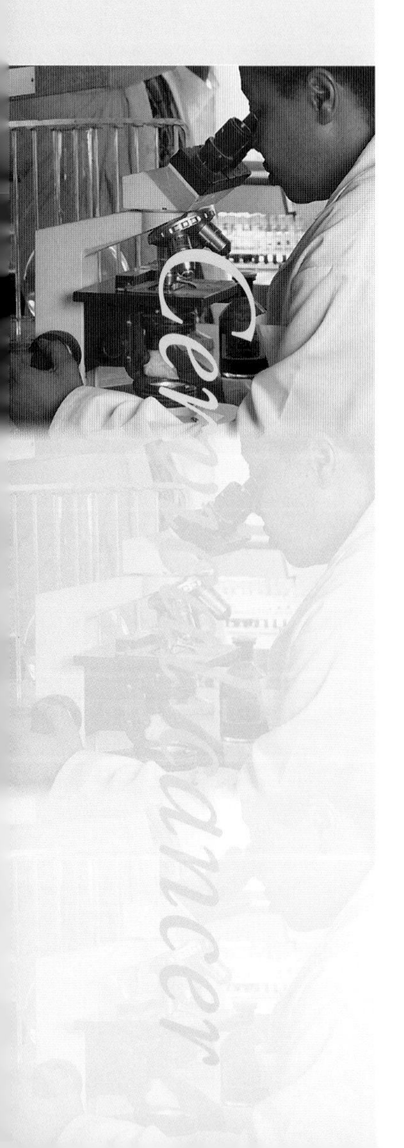

However, 70% of genital HPV infections clear up spontaneously and do not progress to disease. In a minority of women, the infection persists, thereby increasing the risk of pre-malignant cervical lesions which may eventually lead to cervical cancer, usually more than a decade after the original infection. It is estimated that 28–40 million women have pre-malignant HPV infections.

There are an estimated 510 000 new cases of cervical cancer worldwide every year. Of these, 80% occur in developing countries, more than half of them among women in Asia. In 2000, cervical cancer accounted for 288 000 deaths, most of them (272 000) in developing countries.

The disease can be prevented through early diagnosis and treatment. Population-wide screening programmes have dramatically reduced cervical cancer deaths in the developed countries, over the past 50 years. But screening and treatment are very expensive and most low-income countries do not have the resources to introduce population-wide screening programmes which involve regular tests, follow-up and treatment. As a result, few developing countries outside the Americas are able to introduce screening programmes.

While efforts are under way to find an alternative low-cost method for cervical cancer screening in developing countries, a safe and cost-effective vaccine is also needed. The ideal vaccine would prevent both infection with human papillomavirus and the development of cervical cancer among women infected with the virus. Although cervical cancer screening programmes will continue, a vaccine would considerably reduce their cost as fewer women would need to be screened.

Vaccine update

Several candidate vaccines are in the advanced stages of human trials. If one or more of these are successful, it is possible that a vaccine could be available by 2005–6. However, this would still not protect against all HPV strains.

Over 99% of cervical cancers contain HPV DNA, but there are many different HPV types, and immune responses against one may not protect against others. Four specific HPV types cause at least 80% of diagnosed cervical cancers. The ideal vaccine would be a single multivalent vaccine (offering protection against at least four HPV subtypes) that could be used globally.

The most advanced among the different vaccine candidates in development are recombinant protein vaccines against HPV types 16 and 18, which could prevent 50–60% of cervical cancers in both developing and developed countries. Phase II clinical studies are taking place in several countries and large Phase III efficacy trials are planned. Despite the initial emphasis on developed country markets, more than one candidate vaccine will soon be in Phase III testing as a prophylactic vaccine in a developing country context. The US National Cancer Institute (NCI) and several pharmaceutical companies are currently working on these prophylactic vaccine candidates. The NCI has budgeted US$ 20 million for a related project, and investment by the pharmaceutical companies is likely to be

in a similar range. Trials are planned in Brazil, Canada, Colombia, Costa Rica and the United States. Other vaccine candidates include protein-based vaccines and several peptides now being tested in humans as potential therapeutic vaccines. However, these are making slower progress than the candidates mentioned earlier. In addition, live attenuated vectors, such as salmonella, are being investigated as potential second-generation vaccines.

Respiratory syncytial virus (RSV)

Disease burden

RSV is the single most important cause of severe lower respiratory tract infections in infants and young children, involving a wide array of respiratory symptoms including pneumonia and bronchiolitis. Every year there are an estimated 64 million cases of RSV and 160 000 deaths. Most children have been infected by the age of two.

In developed countries, RSV causes annual winter epidemics of acute lower respiratory infection. In the United States alone, it accounts for 18 000 to 75 000 hospital admissions and 90–1900 deaths a year. While few population-based studies have been carried out in developing countries, community-based studies suggest that the highest incidence is in infants less than six months of age, and that approximately two-thirds of RSV-related lower respiratory infections (80% of inpatient cases and 60–70% of outpatient cases) occur in children under two years of age.

Vaccine update

Current vaccine efforts are directed towards the development of a vaccine that incorporates the two RSV serotypes (A and B), or that are directed against their conserved F protein. The development of an RSV vaccine should remain a high priority despite difficulties. The major obstacle is drawn from the experience of earlier clinical trials with formalin-inactivated whole RSV, where children immunized with this vaccine developed a severe form of the disease when exposed to RSV several years later. Therefore, for safety reasons, live attenuated vaccines are considered preferable for immunization of naïve infants although encouraging results are being obtained using purified F protein (PFP) candidate vaccines.

Herpes simplex virus type 2

Disease burden

Herpes simplex virus type 2 (HSV-2) is the most common cause of genital ulcers worldwide. It has been estimated that between 20% and 40% of adults (especially women) have been infected with the virus, with most new infections occurring in persons between 15 and 30 years of age. Once a person has been infected with HSV-2, the virus remains latent in the nerve ganglions of the pelvis, with periodical reactivations which result in painful blisters in the genital area. The virus can be transmitted even if the genital lesions are not apparent.
Although there is no cure for HSV-2, antiviral treatment can shorten or prevent

the development of genital ulcers in an infected person. A significant breakthrough is the recent finding that HSV-2 infections are a major co-factor in HIV infections, increasing the risk of HIV infection by a factor of two to four, depending on the time between the initial HSV-2 infection and exposure to HIV. For this reason, control strategies for HSV-2 need to be incorporated into a comprehensive strategy for HIV prevention, including the development of HSV-2 vaccines.

Vaccine update

A first generation of candidate vaccines against HSV-2 is based on the external glycoproteins of the virus produced by genetic engineering. Although the initial results were not optimal, at least one product showed limited efficacy in a Phase II trial and additional trials are being planned. The newer generation of HSV-2 vaccines are based on replication-defective HSV-2, DNA and epitope-based cocktail vaccines. Two of the challenges to be confronted in the development of HSV-2 vaccines are related to the ability of the virus to establish chronic/latent infections in the presence of anti-HSV-2 immune responses, and the immunological cross-reactivity of HSV-2 with the much more frequent HSV-1, the virus associated with oral herpetic lesions or fever blisters, which complicates the design and analysis of HSV-2 vaccine trials.

Enterotoxigenic Escherichia coli (ETEC)

Disease burden

In developing countries in 2001, diarrhoeal diseases accounted for over 2 million deaths among children under five. Community-based studies have identified *Enterotoxigenic Escherichia coli* (ETEC) as the most frequent cause of episodes of diarrhoeal diseases in this age group, accounting for about 210 million episodes and about 380 000 deaths a year. Most children are infected during the first year of life and the incidence of the disease declines with age.

Although ETEC is usually thought of as a childhood disease, due to its substantially higher incidence in early childhood than in older age groups, almost half of all hospitalized cases of ETEC diarrhoea involve people aged over 10 years, due to the relatively larger population at risk among older age groups. Travellers from developed to developing country settings – including military troops on deployment – are another high risk group for ETEC infection.

Vaccine update

Studies of ETEC infections among children in developing countries suggest that these infections are immunizing – as reflected in the declining rates of ETEC with age – and that immunization against ETEC in early life may be an effective protective strategy.
Because of the antigenic similarity of the B subunits of cholera toxin and ETEC

heat-labile toxin (LT), a recombinant toxin-killed whole cell cholera vaccine was tested in Finnish tourists visiting Morocco. Vaccination prevented 23% of all diarrhoea episodes and 52% of episodes due to ETEC.

The most successful approach, developed by investigators at the University of Goteborg, Sweden, is one in which cholera toxin is combined with five strains of formalin-killed ETEC cells. Phase II studies have found the vaccine to be safe and immunogenic. A pilot efficacy trial of this vaccine in European tourists travelling to developing country destinations found the vaccine provided about 80% protection against ETEC diarrhoea. Phase III trials of vaccine efficacy are ongoing.

The live vaccine approach is being pursued by investigators at the Center for Vaccine Development at the University of Maryland (United States). Their vaccine development strategy is to use live attenuated shigella organisms as vectors for expression of ETEC fimbrial and LT antigens. Such constructs might thereby protect against both shigella and ETEC.

Meanwhile, a new vaccine delivery technology – transcutaneous immunization – involving the use of a patch to deliver vaccine through the skin, has been successfully tested in humans for ETEC vaccine. END Part 3

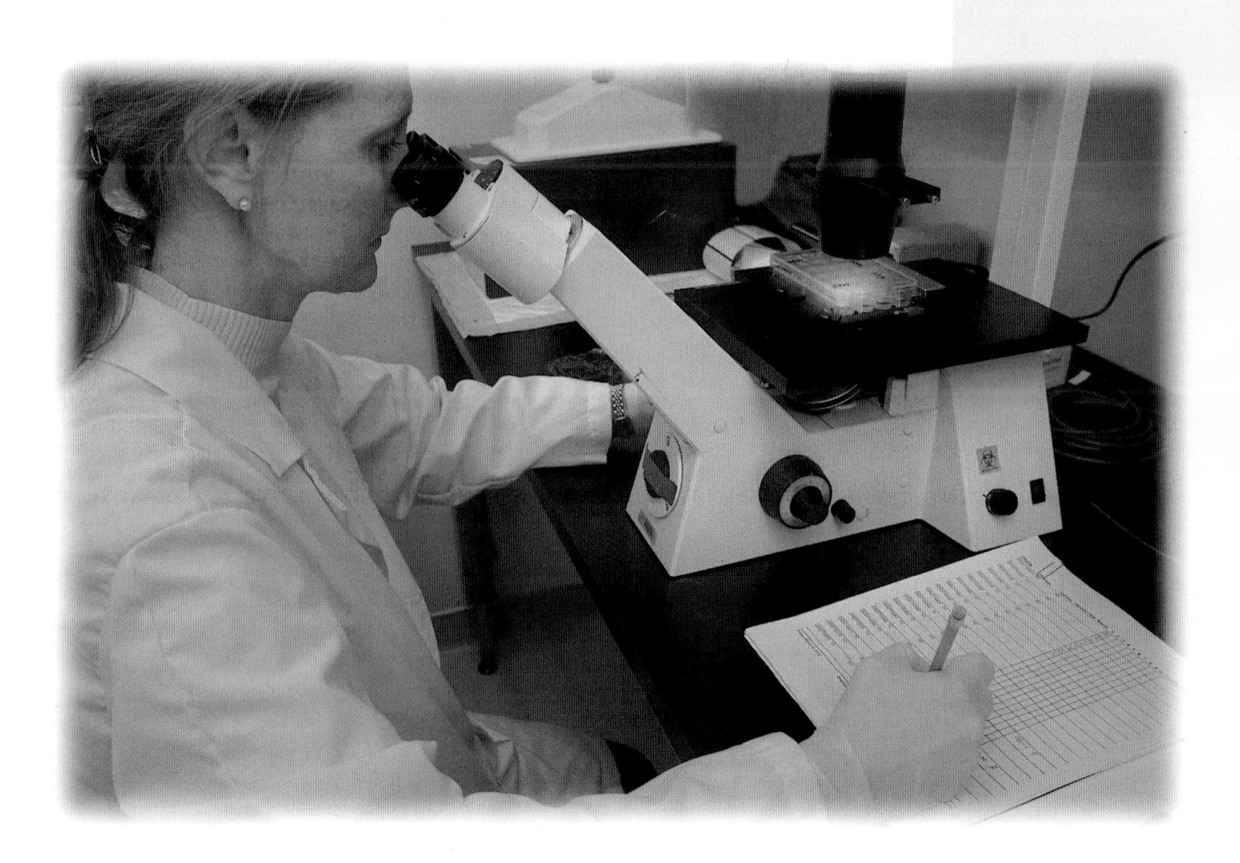

Part 4: Conclusion

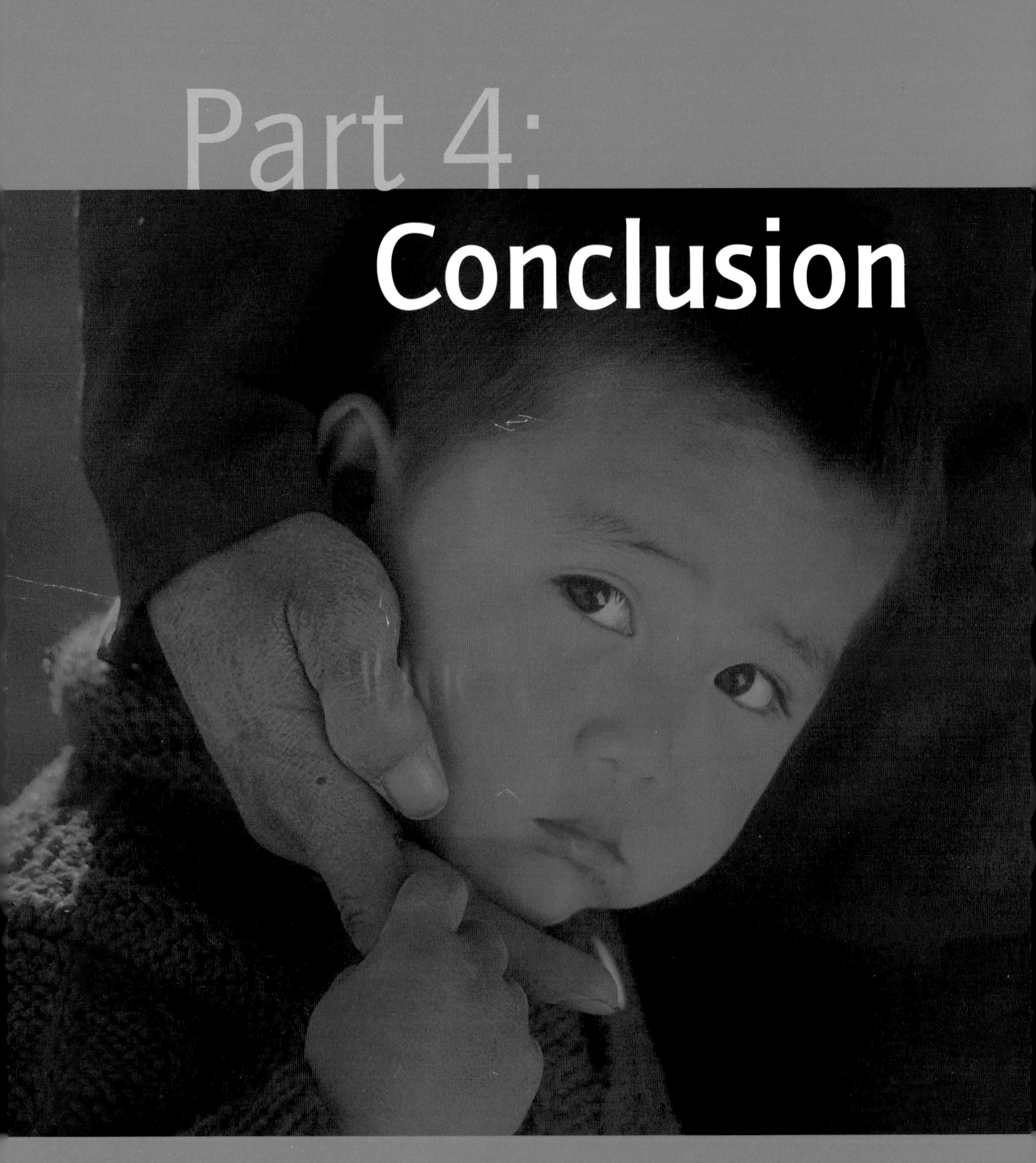

vaccin